ADHD RAISING AN EXPLOSIVE CHILD

The Yell-Free Parenting Strategies to Discipline Even the Most Undisciplined and Unrestrained Child

Ruth Stuart

TABLE OF CONTENTS

INTRODUCTION

Have you ever experienced difficulty with your child's attention span? Have you ever felt like you just couldn't calm them down? Does your child struggle to do tasks that other children their age find easy? Do they become distressed at small things, overstimulated, or bored? There are a lot of things that this could mean. Perhaps your child is oversensitive, on the autism spectrum, or simply is having an emotionally distressing time. But one other explanation is that they are suffering from ADHD.

The good news is that, if this is the case, you are not alone. Many parents across the country have experienced this very same thing. ADHD is very common among teens and adolescents. In fact, as of 2016, over 10% of under-17-year-olds were diagnosed with ADHD, and more specifically just under 8% of under-11-year-olds. Sound high? Now you can start to see how common this condition really is. If you think your child might be experiencing ADHD, or if they have already been diagnosed with ADHD, then you have a wide community of people from which to seek help.

This community spreads around the country, connecting people, and especially parents, who deal with the complications of ADHD. As a modern parent, it's really easy to feel alone. Most parents both work outside the home—many taking on long and stressful hours—and spend a lot of time shuttling their kids around to various after school activities. It can be hard to maintain a social life and be able to ascertain what kinds of things other parents and children are going through. When your child is acting unruly and testing every bit of patience you have, it can be easy to feel like you're doing something wrong, like *why me*. But if you really look at the statistics, you will realize that many parents are feeling exactly the same thing.

Luckily, because of the prevalence of ADHD, there has been a lot of research done about it—including symptoms, effects, and treatments. There are also many support groups and online communities formed for both people with ADHD and for parents of children who have ADHD. Once your child is formally diagnosed, you can start to take advantage of this research and resources in order to start building more resilience as a family and helping your child to be the best that they can be.

The first step though is, of course, to educate yourself. In order to support your child through their ADHD journey, you need to be as informed as possible of the ins and outs of the condition. ADHD is one of the most commonly misunderstood conditions in the world. Many people assume that a lack of attention span is the only symptom of ADHD, but there are actually many more than that, with even the attention span symptom being more complicated than most people believe. When something is widely misunderstood, then it can be really challenging to deal with it in the real world. People might have offensive stereotypes in mind when dealing with you or your child, which can be challenging to face. But education is the best tool in helping to recalibrate people's minds towards acceptance.

You yourself might even have some stereotypes in mind about ADHD. This might have caused you to doubt your child or be reluctant to get them diagnosed. You might think that people with ADHD will never go far in life, never really accomplish their goals or be successful. You might worry that being diagnosed with ADHD will make people see your child differently or make your child see themselves differently. But the world is changing, and there is no need to think these things anymore. Holding beliefs like this can prevent you from getting your child the help they need and, most importantly, accepting them for who they are.

One factor that can really skew people's understanding of children with ADHD is the fact that all people, especially children, are different and develop at different rates. Your child might exhibit a unique set of ADHD symptoms which are wholly unique from other children, and their symptoms might even change over time. However, this does not mean their symptoms have gone away. This is a crucial aspect of understanding ADHD: It is not a curable condition, only a treatable one. Therefore, if your child starts losing some of their symptoms, they are likely growing into a different manifestation of their ADHD. With help, they can mitigate their symptoms and work towards accommodating their differences.

In this book, you will find a comprehensive guide to parenting an ADHD child. We will be showing you all that you need to know to support your child through their ADHD journey. In the first chapter, we will cover the basics of ADHD as a condition, outlining types, symptoms, and different manifestations for different demographics. Next, in Chapter 2, we will talk about the neuroscience of ADHD, helping you to understand the ways in which your child's brain is different. After that, Chapter 3 will discuss how your role as a parent figures into your child's ADHD diagnosis. Following this chapter, we will take a deep dive into the prioritizing of your own mental health in the midst of dealing with your child's. Chapter 5 will then pivot to talking more specifically about how to deal with your child's inevitable outbursts, teaching you how to manage conflict and support them through that experience.

Then, in the sixth chapter, we will talk about more long-term preventative measures you can take for developing emotional regulation in your child. Chapter 7 will deal with the development of healthy habits in the home, helping you to create an environment that encourages self-regulation and accommodates your child's needs. Chapter 8 will then discuss the use of executive function in forming more sustainable life skills for your kids. After that, we will talk about bonding with your child and helping them to open up to you, especially about issues related to their ADHD. Communication is key when it comes to these relationships and is thus one of the most important components of your child's ADHD recovery journey. And in the final chapter, we will talk about the ways in which your child's ADHD can actually be used to their advantage, as a superpower! Through all these chapters, you will get a window into the many ins and outs of parenting an ADHD child. By the end of the book, you should have the confidence you need to start supporting your child and leading them towards the path to success!

CHAPTER 1:

GETTING TO KNOW ADHD

Before you can help your child, you need to learn about their condition. Understanding what is going on with them is integral to being able to make sense of their behavior. If you are uninformed about ADHD, you will never be able to give your children the attention they really need to thrive. Knowing what's going on with them is going to really help you in the long run, skyrocketing the both of you towards more understanding and acceptance of one another. It will also help them not to feel too alone and gain the support they need to thrive.

In this chapter, we will be looking at the basic features of ADHD, educating you on all the essential things you need to know about your child's condition. We will start with a basic definition of what ADHD really is, showing you the major signs and symptoms. Then, we will talk about different types of ADHD and how they might manifest in different people. After that, we will debunk some of the most common myths and misconceptions about ADHD that people tend to have. And to finish, we will compare the difference between how ADHD manifests in children versus in adults. By the end of the chapter, you should be well-versed in the essential qualities of ADHD.

What Is ADHD?

So first of all, what exactly *is* ADHD? Well, ADHD stands for attention deficit hyperactivity disorder. It is also sometimes, or formerly, known as ADD—attention deficit disorder. It is characterized by irregular attention span and hyperactivity. Irregular attention span means the inability to focus on certain tasks, while hyper-focusing on others. This can often lead to procrastination, unfinished projects, and losing track of time very easily. Hyperactivity is characterized by an inability to sit still and a constant sense of urgency. These are the two main sides of ADHD that will be diagnosed if and when your child sees a psychiatrist. Here, we will talk about some of the main features of ADHD.

Neurodivergence

ADHD falls under the umbrella of something called "neurodivergence." In base terms, being neurodivergent means having any kind of condition that affects cognitive function. The roots of the word neuro, meaning brain, and divergent, meaning different from the norm, signifies having different cognitive processes than the general population. This can come in many forms, such as difficulty concentrating, reading emotions, holding down jobs, interacting with others, etc. Many of these things mean that people with neurodivergent conditions will have significantly more struggles in life than those who do not suffer from these conditions. There are varying degrees of seriousness to the conditions that fall under this descriptor, and some might even be caused by physical conditions. All of these conditions will require unique accommodations, and so, they will have completely different experiences with both symptoms and treatment. However, the label of neurodivergent helps psychologists and facilitators to categorize people who may struggle to perform school, work, or social tasks.

With the right accommodations, neurodivergent people can create environments that are suitable for them and start to perform better at certain tasks, even excel. In fact, neurodivergence can be a debilitating thing, but it can also be a superpower. Just as we will talk about in the last chapter of this book, there are many things that people with neurodivergence actually excel at over others. Thus, there are also things to celebrate about neurodivergence. In this section, we will talk a bit more about neurodivergence and how it relates to ADHD.

What Conditions Fall Under Neurodivergence?

Almost any mental illness or disability can be considered neurodivergence, since your brain is functioning differently from other people. However, there is a clear list of conditions that are most commonly associated with the term neurodivergent. Here are the generally-defined neurodivergent conditions:

- Autism Spectrum Disorder (ASD)
- ADHD
- Dyslexia
- Dyspraxia
- Down Syndrome
- Obsessive Compulsive Disorder (OCD)
- Sensory Processing Disorder
- Bipolar Disorder
- Anxiety Disorder
- Tourette's Syndrome

This list is quite a diverse one. Perhaps, when reading it, you felt a pang of fear for your child, since there are some very serious conditions on this list. But there is no need to worry. Just because these conditions might have similar qualities does not mean your child is necessarily more susceptible to them, especially genetic disorders present from birth like Down's syndrome. The purpose of categorizing this list is to show that there are several conditions known to psychology that can have a significant effect on your ability to function and your cognitive process. Something that a lot of neurodivergent people have in common is a tendency towards overstimulation. Because the world is not organized around the particular processing needs of neurodivergent brains, neurodivergent people tend to find the outside world scary or too much for them and can easily become overstimulated, even in situations you might not think they would. This may be a contributing factor to their high functionality among online spaces, which can provide as mediation for some of the overstimulating symptoms of neurodivergence. If you notice that your child tends to become easily overstimulated or has an easier time communicating with people digitally, then these are common generalized neurodivergence symptoms, of which their ADHD is the most specific branch.

Neurodivergent Versus Neurotypical

So, if people with ADHD, ASD, OCD, etc. are neurodivergent, then what is everyone else? Generally, psychologists refer to those without particular psychological needs as "neurotypical." While neurotypicals might have other conditions, they, for the most part, have brains which function according to the way society is structured. Neurotypical people don't often struggle in mainstream situations, tend to respond well to standardized testing, and don't require a lot of specialized accommodations to

10

function in society. Though this dichotomy may sound harsh, it is important to note that a major advantage neurotypical people have over neurodivergent people is simply that there are more of them, and therefore, the world is structured around them. Most schooling is catered to the neurotypical brain, and most social interactions assume a neurotypical thinking pattern in other people. Though there are legitimate struggles to many neurodivergent conditions, a huge portion of the struggle is simply battling a world explicitly designed for neurotypicals with little to no consideration for neurodivergent ways of being. As more awareness is raised for these conditions, life for neurodivergent people is becoming a lot easier. Diagnosis and access to accommodations is thus one of the most important things for neurotypical people in their journey, helping to make their world a little less neurotypical and a little more suited to their unique set of needs.

ADHD Symptoms

There are as many ADHD symptoms as there are sufferers. That is to say, there are numerous symptoms, many of which you might not even recognize as such. There might be some things your child does that you don't even realize are because of their ADHD. When perusing the following list of symptoms, reflect on whether you think your child may be exhibiting these behaviors. There are two main categories to ADHD symptoms, as we mentioned before, each with their own set of symptoms. However, if your child has ADHD, it's likely they are experiencing symptoms from across the board.

Attention Deficit Symptoms

- Becoming easily distracted
- Difficulty with organization and deadlines
- Switching frequently between tasks
- Particularly struggling with tasks that require a lot of time commitment or that are tedious
- Frequently making careless mistakes, especially at schoolwork
- Losing things all the time

Hyperactivity Symptoms

- Excessive talking
- Constant fidgeting
- Impulsive actions
- Frequently interrupting others
- Careless about safety, often engaging in risky behavior
- Trouble waiting their turn

If your child is showing any of these signs — and especially if they show a lot of them — then it is likely they are experiencing ADHD. Many of these symptoms can cause your child difficulty in life—both in school and social situations. Difficulty concentrating or sitting still might make it difficult for them to do schoolwork, and excessive talking or interrupting might cause other children to avoid them. If your child is experiencing these things, then look into whether ADHD might be behind it all.

The good news is that many of these symptoms are manageable, and your child will be well on their way towards mitigating these behaviors with the right treatment. We will talk more in the next section about what happens when one only shows symptoms of one of the types of ADHD.

Types of ADHD

If you read the list of symptoms in the last section, but only seemed to resonate with one set of them, then your child might be experiencing a distinctive type of ADHD. In medical terms, there are actually three types of ADHD: inattentive, hyperactive, or combined. Although all three are considered ADHD, they each have distinctive qualities that mean that they will have different experiences from one another. Here, we will look at the main differences between these three types of ADHD.

Inattentive ADHD

When you picture someone with ADHD, you might picture a child staring out the window, unable to focus on their work. Although it is a bit more complex than that, there is some truth to this image. Those with inattentive ADHD primarily struggle with tasks related to attention. Generally, an inability to pay attention tends to be the popular conception of this condition, but there is another side to it. While those with ADHD do have trouble concentrating a lot of the time, they also tend towards something called hyper-focusing. Hyper-focusing occurs when someone is so focused on a specific task that they completely lose track of all else, sometimes even forgetting to eat or go to the bathroom! If you have been thinking: *Well, my child can't have ADHD, they sit up in their room and draw for hours!* That is actually hyper-focusing, which can be characteristic of ADHD just as much as struggling with focus. Those with inattentive ADHD simply have trouble regulating their attention, focusing intently on things while they are interested, and being completely unable to focus when they are not. It can get particularly difficult when the full extent of this range of focus is experienced towards the same thing, and they lose interest and abandon their projects never to be picked up again!

Hyperactive ADHD

The other image of ADHD you might have in your head is a child ceaselessly fidgeting in their seat, unable to sit still. This is the main symptom of hyperactive ADHD. This is the much more outwardly obvious form of ADHD, but there are still many symptoms that are not so obviously connected to ADHD. The kind of social unawareness that goes along with the constant speaking and interruptions might not initially be identified as ADHD to the less keen eye, but make no mistake that this is a telltale symptom. Nevertheless, this type of ADHD remains more commonly diagnosed than inattentive ADHD, simply because it is more outwardly intrusive.

Combined ADHD

The final type of ADHD is combined ADHD. As you can probably guess from the name, combined ADHD is a mix of some of the most integral aspects of the two. If you were connecting all of the symptoms in the last section to your child, then it is highly likely that they are experiencing combined ADHD. This condition will involve both the qualities of inattentive and hyperactive ADHD.

Identifying Symptoms and Types

As we have mentioned throughout the last two sections, everyone's experience of ADHD is different. Your child's

ADHD symptoms are going to look very different from another child's. What this means is that identifying what exactly is going on with your child can be very hard. You might not have the typical kicking-and-screaming or head-in-the-clouds ADHD that you have seen depicted in the media. Instead, your child might exhibit only a few, more obscure symptoms, leading you astray. Misdiagnosis is also very common with ADHD. Your child may have been diagnosed with ASD or OCD or even a generalized learning disability, when what they really have is ADHD. Diagnosing these kinds of conditions is extremely challenging, and only professionals can actually do it properly, but it's important for you to understand how diagnosis works so that you can help your child get diagnosed. In this section, we are going to talk about the different ways ADHD manifests and how you can identify it as such.

Differing Symptoms: Case Studies

As previously mentioned, your child's experience with ADHD might be different from another's. There are plenty of different symptoms that might combine with one another or interact with specific personalities or life situations and thus manifest differently. The wide variation that can be seen amongst those who suffer from ADHD means that there are a lot of misdiagnoses or people who go underdiagnosed. In this section, we will review some more specific hypothetical case studies of different combinations of symptoms that might interact with one another to form a unique ADHD personality. Through these (hypothetical) examples, you will be able to see how ADHD is different among different personality types.

Case Study #1: The Chatty Cathy

Let's say you have a girl who is eight years old. She is very well-spoken, often getting compliments that she is mature for her age based on her vocabulary. However, she often gets in trouble at school for constantly chatting to her friends, talking over the teacher, and generally interrupting lessons. What's more, she never seems to perform in school, despite her obvious intelligence. She feels that verbalization is the only way she can really express herself, and thus does not do well on tests, nor can she restrain herself from showing off her vocal skills at every turn. It might be that this girl is actually experiencing ADHD, just with a focus on the verbal sides of hyperactivity. You might not recognize it as such, since she doesn't fit the stereotypical symptoms, but it is highly likely. If she were to get a diagnosis and accommodations from teachers who could play to her talents, perhaps offering her oral tests or more opportunities to incorporate conversation into learning, she would be able to boost her grades and start reaping some of the recognition she deserves!

Case Study #2: The Fidget Master

Our next case study is a child who seems to be constantly fidgeting. They are generally not super athletic or rambunctious, but they are just always shaking their leg or tapping their toes. You notice that this seems to actually help them concentrate. They can't seem to get anything done unless their body is moving in some way. They show increased productivity or attention span when they have a fidget toy or a small bicycle pedal under their seats. You wonder if they just have a lot of energy to burn off, but this can actually also be a sign of ADHD. Many people with ADHD struggle with chronic understimulation, a condition wherein they feel like they don't have enough to do or that their minds are constantly bored. Even if they seemingly have a task, such as a homework assignment or just watching a movie, they still don't feel stimulated enough. It sounds counter-intuitive, but for these people actually having more to do makes it easier to concentrate. Things like toe tapping or fidgeting can help engage the child's body as well as their mind, helping them to regulate their levels of stimulation and actually concentrate better. If you notice that your child is a chronic fidgeter or always needs to be thoroughly engaged in a task, then they might actually have ADHD.

Case Study #3: The Hyperfocuser

Imagine you have a child who is a prolific artist. They are constantly sketching in their notebook, developing their drawing skills. Often, they will become so engaged in their work that they actually cannot pay attention to anything else. You call their name from downstairs and they seem not to hear you, or rather you attempt to engage them in another activity and they seem not to be able to pull themselves away. They might even become so absorbed that they forget to eat or go to the bathroom, completely losing track of time. You might feel conflicted about being frustrated with them over this. After all, they're pursuing their hobbies and doing something productive. But they just don't seem to be able to manage their time and often end up forgetting important things like homework assignments or chores. Well, this can actually be a sign of ADHD, even though they seem to be concentrating very well. One of the biggest misconceptions about ADHD is that people with the condition cannot focus on anything. Hyper-focusing is actually a very common symptom and can lead to many of the same consequences as lack of focus. If you find that your child often focuses on things to the exclusion of all else and absolutely cannot be roused, they might actually have a focusing disorder, such as ADHD.

ADHD *in Girls Vs Boys*

As we know, ADHD presents differently in everyone, but there are often trends amongst different demographics affecting how their ADHD manifests. Girls and boys often show their ADHD in very different ways. Boys are also far more likely to receive a diagnosis for ADHD—as much as three times more likely than girls (Kinman, 2012). However, this disparity is not necessarily biological. There is no evidence showing that there are any neurological differences between girls and boys, and certainly none powerful enough to affect something as major as ADHD susceptibility. ADHD is not more common in boys, it is just more commonly-diagnosed. Likewise, ADHD is not different in boys and girls, but the ways in which boys and girls are treated in the world, as well as narratives from themselves and others about their own behavior, means that they will find different outlets for their ADHD. In this section, we will explore how symptoms tend to differ between boys and girls, investigating why this might be the case, and exploring the ways in which you can identify ADHD in a more diverse way.

Typical Boy ADHD Symptoms

Boys are the stereotypical ADHD sufferers. Most of the behavior we associate with ADHD—disruptive moving and talking, roughhousing, hyperactive behavior, etc.—are also considered to be typically "boyish" behaviors. Because of cultural "boys will be boys" narratives, we tend to allow boys to express more roughness or loudness and reprimand them less for this behavior. As such, boys with ADHD have a tendency to lean into their hyperactivity especially. They have more outwardly-presenting symptoms because they are more expected to act in that way. They might even experience social capital for acting out in that way; being the roughest and the loudest might actually earn them respect from other boys, who might see this as a sign of power. Again, this can make them lean even more into it, with their ADHD helping them feel more aligned with traditional masculinity. But because of this more extreme expression, they tend to be more frequently flagged by teachers. Educators might find this behavior extremely disruptive to class time, especially since ADHD boys can act as ringleaders to other boys, siphoning authority from the teachers. As there are more outward symptoms of boys' ADHD, it is more easily identified, and thus, boys are more likely to be diagnosed. Here are some of the most common symptoms associated with ADHD in boys:

- inattentiveness or outright ignoring
- frequent interruptions, especially of authority figures
- impulsive behavior
- attention-seeking behavior
- hyperactivity, either kinetic (running, jumping, etc.) or aggressive (fighting, kicking, etc.)

- excessive talking

If you notice that your son is expressing many of these symptoms, it is likely that he is experiencing ADHD. However, it is not always that clear-cut. Sometimes, girls will express these kinds of symptoms as well, and sometimes, boys will express some of the more "girly" symptoms. It all depends on their personality, their culture, and environment they were raised in. Don't worry if your child is not displaying the symptoms associated with their gender; this is just a basic guideline of averages. Nevertheless, it is important to understand the diversity of symptoms possible.

Typical Girl ADHD Symptoms

When girls have ADHD, it can be a lot harder to tell. Behavior like running, fighting, and interrupting are not typically feminine traits. It is likely that girls with ADHD had these symptoms stamped out of them from a very young age due to the harsher restrictions around how girls are meant to act in the world. As a result, many girls internalize their ADHD symptoms. While boys' symptoms are external—meaning that they are typically directed at or are significantly disruptive to others—girls' symptoms are typically directed at themselves. They will be far less noticeable for this reason, because girls become much better at hiding their symptoms and directing them inwards. So, instead of getting in a fight with someone on the playground, a girl with ADHD might withdraw completely, perhaps directing that aggression towards herself, worsening her self-esteem. In fact, girls with ADHD tend to have chronically low self-esteem for this very reason. They will often be very frustrated with themselves for not being able to meet expectations and thus act with anger toward themselves, rather than others. This can lead to lifelong issues with performance anxiety and self-worth, which is why it is so important for girls to get diagnosed and treated for ADHD as soon as possible. Here are some of the most common ADHD symptoms in girls:

- social withdrawal or extreme extroversion, frequently chatting with classmates when they should be working
- difficulty focusing
- being labeled "dreamy" or "spacey"
- low self-esteem
- verbal bullying or teasing
- anxiety
- low academic performance

As you can see, these symptoms are quite different from the typical boy symptoms of ADHD. This is a testament to how much environment and circumstances can change the way that ADHD works in the brain. Of these symptoms, there are two distinctive types that stand out. You may have noticed that some of these symptoms are contradictory, with some girls tending to be very socially withdrawn and some being very extroverted. This is generally the dichotomy that girls with ADHD fall into: the "dreamer" and the "chatty Cathy." These two archetypes represent ways that ADHD can fit into stereotypically feminine behavior. Some girls choose to be more withdrawn, often favoring reading or art, not being able to make friends, and yet still performing poorly academically. These girls might have a special interest where they excel—similar to the ADHD phenomenon of hyper-focusing—but then perform poorly elsewhere, such as being at an extremely high reading level, but struggling with other subjects in school.

The chatty Cathy archetype might seem completely the opposite, a social butterfly. She seems to have millions of friends and will prioritize those relationships (and talking) over all else. She might struggle to stay quiet in class, needing to vocalize her every thought. If she is bolder, or has more self-esteem issues, this can slide into ringleader or bullying behavior. She might be a bit of a queen bee, encouraging others to act out along with her and punishing those who hurt her feelings. She might even talk back to teachers. But because both of these behaviors, although cause for concern, don't raise the same (especially physical) disruptions as boys, much of it will slip under the radar. Helping your daughter to get the proper care she needs for her ADHD will help to curb these behaviors and turn them into something positive instead. Again, there is not necessarily such a stark divide, as boys and girls can engage in both behaviors, but it is important to know, especially if you have a daughter, that there are a specific set of symptoms that she is more prone to due to her gender.

ADHD in Children Vs Adults

Throughout this chapter, we have mainly discussed the role of ADHD in children, but did you know that adults can also have ADHD? ADHD is actually considered a lifelong condition. There is no actual cure, only treatments and accommodations, and so if a child is diagnosed with ADHD, they will have it (in some form) for life, and if an adult is diagnosed with ADHD, it means they also had it as a child. But just as people don't stay the same in general throughout their entire lives, people's ADHD also doesn't stay the same. Adults have wildly different lives than children, and thus, their ADHD will manifest very differently. In this section, we will talk about some of the factors that change from childhood to adulthood which affect ADHD, for better or for worse.

Responsibility

Obviously, the biggest difference between children and adults is their levels of responsibility. Other than perhaps a few after school chores, children have next to no responsibility at all. If they fail at something, they are at no risk of losing their home and safety, assuming they are in a non-abusive home situation with good parents. Children with ADHD thus face far fewer consequences for their actions. Parents and teachers are likely doing all that they can to help the child with ADHD, whereas most adults won't get that from most of the people they interact with in the adult world. As much as their boss, partner, or other people in their life might care about them, they are not tasked with being an ADHD support person and thus the adult with ADHD is more or less on their own, except perhaps for their therapist or very close loved ones. Undiagnosed people are often met with a rude awakening when they enter the adult world. Failing to hand things in might have gotten them a slap on the wrist in school, it gets them fired in the adult world. But because they have not learned about their own condition and gained the tools for how to manage it, they are completely on their own in a world of increased responsibility. Diagnosed people, on the other hand, especially those who have received very high-quality treatment, will be able to manage their symptoms to be able to function in the adult world. They will know the kinds of coping mechanisms that work for them, the accommodations they need to ask for and give themselves, and the limits of their condition. The children who receive treatment will have a much easier time integrating into the adult world simply because they have the tools to take on more responsibility. For this reason of increased responsibility and decreased support, it is imperative that children get diagnosed early so that they develop the tools to help themselves in the world at a young age.

Relationships

When you become an adult, the relationships in your life change fundamentally. You go from being primarily dependent on others to having others depend on you, your relationships becoming more two-sided and sometimes even one-sided for others, especially if you become a parent. People with ADHD tend to struggle with relationships, with many children struggling to make friends. This will continue into adult life if left unchecked and can lead to insecure adult relationships, especially romantic ones. Adults with untreated ADHD have been known to flit from relationship to relationship, unable to commit to any one person for a long time. That tendency to get bored easily and have trouble persevering at something past the initial honeymoon stage can lead to very unstable adult relationships. Having insecure or avoidant attachment styles can be particularly devastating as a parent, since children need extremely consistent, unconditional love and care. If an ADHD parent becomes disinterested in their child, it can be disastrous for the child's development. For these reasons, getting the help you need as early on in life as possible is integral to avoiding those dangerous pitfalls in relationships that come with untreated adult ADHD.

Autonomy

Finally, the adult world involves a lot more autonomy, which can be both a blessing and a curse for those with ADHD. While children live heavily structured lives, with almost everything they do being dictated and scheduled out for them, with very little room for their input or freedom, adults have much more control over their lives. In terms of career, you generally can choose what kind of hours you want to work, what kind of environment you want to work in, and what kind of work you want to do, unlike school, which is essentially the same for everyone. In your free time, you don't have any parents telling you what to do, so you can do anything you want, financially permitting. On one hand, this increased freedom means that adults with ADHD can accommodate their condition much better than children can. Many adults with ADHD choose to do freelance work or work from home so as to mitigate some of the anxiety they might feel around restrictive or overstimulating environments and strict schedules. They might also have more power to request certain working conditions and to take time off when they need it. However, on the other hand, increased autonomy can leave a lot of room for things like procrastination, understimulation, and general lack of productivity. Adults with ADHD might find that they aren't able to concentrate as well as they did in school because they have no one telling them what to do and are expected to take more initiative. Thus, many people with ADHD find adult freedom and autonomy to be a mixed blessing, helping them to accommodate their condition, but also taking away structure that might have helped them stay on track. But if they have received adequate treatment, they should be able to reap the positives from autonomy, knowing the accommodations they need, and experience none of the drawbacks by having adequate accommodations.

Myths and Misconceptions

Like most disorders, there are a fair amount of misconceptions people might have about ADHD as a condition. Miseducation and offensive stereotypes about the condition are rampant, and there are plenty of opportunities for incomprehension. This kind of lack of information can actually have very dire consequences on your child's access to resources, as we talked about in the introduction. Thus, it is very important to be aware of the misconceptions you or others might have about your child's condition. Here are some of the most common myths out there about ADHD.

Myth #1: ADHD Is Overdiagnosed

You might hear this said by a lot of people, especially those that have a lot of mistrust in institutions like psychiatry or pharmaceuticals. They might say things like "ADHD was designed to put kids on drugs" or "They diagnose kids with too many things these days." This couldn't be further from the truth. Let the myth be busted: ADHD is a real disorder affecting millions of people and which is actually routinely underdiagnosed, not overdiagnosed. There are many people, children and adults alike in this world living with underdiagnosed ADHD. This means that they think that there is something wrong with them and are unable to seek the kind of support they need. All that happens when we under-diagnose ADHD is that those suffering lack support and accommodations, and we are all the worse for it.

Myth #2: All People With ADHD Are Medicated

One of the major components to Myth #1 is that ADHD is designed to sell drugs and that too many people are medicated these days. While many people with ADHD, including children, do take medication to help manage their symptoms, it is not necessarily the only solution. Many of the treatments available for ADHD involve no drugs at all, simply accommodations from schools and support from therapists and loved ones. Having an independent education plan where your child has more lenient deadlines or a quieter workspace might be all they need to keep their symptoms in check. Even amongst those children who do go on medication, these other accommodations will still play a key role in their treatment. Therefore, not all ADHD sufferers are medicated, and even those who are still have other components to their treatment. Whether you want to use medication to help manage your child's symptoms is completely up to you and your family. No doctor will pressure you into doing so and thus you have the choice to make completely on your own.

Myth #3: ADHD Is Caused by Poor Parenting

This is one myth that you yourself might hold and which might be seriously inhibiting you from getting your child diagnosed. You might be experiencing a lot of shame around your child's ADHD diagnosis or symptoms. You might be wondering what you did wrong or how you could have parented them differently to make sure that this didn't happen. But the good news is that there is no clear link between parenting style and the development of ADHD. You can rest assured that you didn't do anything wrong to get your child diagnosed. However, there is a link between parenting style and response to treatment. The biggest test for you as an ADHD parent is how well you support your child through their journey. If you deny your child's ADHD, prevent them from getting treatment,

31

and refuse to acknowledge your preconceived notions, you will be setting your child up for failure. However, if you are highly accepting, educate yourself, and work hard to facilitate your child's treatment and accommodations, then you will be helping them on the path to recovery.

Myth #4: Only Boys Have ADHD

If you are picturing a boy every time we talk about ADHD examples, then you are not alone. Many people associate ADHD as a condition with boys specifically. This is because many of the behaviors associated with ADHD are also associated with typical boyish behavior. In school-age children, boys are generally thought to play outside and roughhouse, while girls are generally thought to read more and perform better in school. These gendered expectations mean that girls tend to mask their ADHD much better than boys, often slipping under the radar when it comes to flagging children for ADHD. For this reason, boys are more commonly diagnosed with the condition. As a result, most people believe that boys have ADHD at much higher rates than girls do, which couldn't be further from the truth. In actuality, there is no clear gender bias when it comes to ADHD. If you have a daughter, she might not seem like the typical picture of someone with ADHD. However, it is likely that she is either exhibiting unique symptoms or is very good at masking her disorder. If this is the case, then you need to make sure that you are giving her the same attention that you would a son. The gendered bias of ADHD is, put simply, only in the minds of people, not proven in reality.

CHAPTER 2:

UNDERSTANDING YOUR CHILD'S BRAIN AND BEHAVIORS

ADHD is fundamentally a brain disorder. It actually affects the very chemistry of the brain, reading completely differently on brain scans. The conditions of ADHD will be greatly affected by the conditions of the brain and vice versa. For you to understand what your child is going through, it is imperative to understand what is going on in their brain. So much of what is happening to them is outside of their control and happening below the surface. It is likely that they have no idea what is going on in there either and so it is your responsibility as the parent to do the research and learn about what is happening to them neurologically. You don't necessarily have to have a degree in neuroscience, but gaining a base knowledge of the brain as an organ, and specifically the ADHD brain, can greatly help you in dealing with the illness and helping your child through it. In this chapter, we will talk all about ADHD and the brain, showing you all the many ways in which it can be affected. First, we will talk about the child's brain. As this is a book not just about ADHD, but more specifically about childhood ADHD, you need to understand how children's brains specifically work. Then, we will talk about how brains with ADHD compare to brains without ADHD. After that, we will discuss the important connection between the mind and the body, demonstrating how important physical health and wellness is to ADHD recovery. By the end of this chapter, you should have a thorough knowledge of the way in which ADHD is working in your child's mind.

The Child's Brain

Before you can understand the ADHD child's mind, you need to be able to understand the way that a child's brain works, as well as the brain in general. There are specific ways in which the brain develops that can interact with ADHD in unique ways to form a complex series of developments. The child's brain is, in essence, underdeveloped. It does not have the same features as an adult brain and thus is both more susceptible to influence, but also better at learning. In this section, we will talk about two distinctive aspects of the child's brain. The first will deal with the parts of the brain and how they develop throughout childhood and adolescence. The second part will talk about how ADHD can influence and interact with this development to form a different adult brain.

Parts of the Brain

The brain has many different aspects to it. Although it might seem like just a big pile of goop, there are millions of cells, chemicals, and connections working tirelessly within your brain in order to perform all the functions it needs to throughout the day. With children in particular, the brain is not only performing these functions, but growing at the same time. Thus, the child's brain, with all its aspects, is going to look completely different from the adult's brain. Here, we will look at some specific parts of the brain, how they work, and how they develop over time.

The Prefrontal Cortex

Perhaps the starkest difference between child and adult minds is the prefrontal cortex. The prefrontal cortex is a part of the brain located in the frontal lobe, just behind your forehead. It is responsible for your highest rational thinking. Things like long-term planning, identity, higher decision making, and socialization are all the job of the prefrontal cortex. In Freudian terms, you might call the prefrontal cortex the 'ego' or the 'superego,' regulating social and individual behavior and allowing us to mitigate our urges and desires with rational thinking. As you can see, many of these things are qualities associated with maturity or adulthood. After all, children and teenagers are notorious for lacking long-term planning skills or strong senses of identity. This isn't by accident—the prefrontal cortex is one of the last parts of the brain to fully develop. Thus, the prefrontal cortex has an integral role in the development of the child's brain into the adult's brain.

So what does this mean for your child? Well, it means that they very likely are going to struggle with the main functions of the prefrontal cortex, at no fault of their own. They will have trouble associating consequences with actions, especially ones that are long-term. This is why many parents have to impose short-term consequences on certain actions so that children can avoid the long-term consequences that they have trouble visualizing. For example, an adult knows that if they don't brush their teeth, they will get cavities. But because cavities can take weeks or months to develop, a child cannot really grasp that far ahead. Thus, they need a short-term incentive to brush their teeth, such as being threatened with punishment or promised a reward. The prefrontal cortex continues to develop well into your 20s, not fully developing until the age of 25, and so your child will continue to struggle with these things up until this age at least.

When it comes to ADHD, the prefrontal cortex, as a regulating organ, is essential to helping them manage their symptoms as they get older. However, the development of the prefrontal cortex should not be mistaken for simply "growing out" of ADHD. Coincidentally, many of the things that children with underdeveloped prefrontal cortexes struggle with are also ADHD symptoms. And while many children do grow out of things like difficulty regulating their emotions and behavior, people with ADHD do not. We will talk more in the next section about how ADHD specifically affects the prefrontal cortex as well as its development.

Neurotransmitters

The brain is full of chemicals called neurotransmitters. These chemicals help with the transmission of information and can affect mood, energy levels, and many other functions of the mind and body. We all have a collection of chemicals in our brain which forms our unique brain chemistry. There are many brain chemicals, but the most important ones are:

Dopamine

Also known as the "happy chemical," dopamine is responsible for short-term boosts in mood. It's what you feel when you bite into a chocolate bar, ride a roller coaster, or have any other intense experience where you feel a rush. Dopamine also plays a central role in your reward system, incentivizing you to continue behaviors that pump dopamine into your system. On one hand, dopamine is great because it feels good and can help you develop great behaviors, but on the other hand, it can also cause addiction if hijacked in the wrong way. Children in particular respond well to dopamine, because they are so apt to short-term reward. When a child becomes too reliant on dopamine, it can risk their ability to self-regulate. Children thus need to learn to mitigate their reliance on dopamine-inducing stimuli so that they can begin to develop long-term planning and rewards. Dopamine can also be a powerful brain chemical to use to help treat ADHD, but we will cover that in a later section.

Serotonin

The sister brain chemical to dopamine, serotonin is known as the long-term happy chemical. It helps with things like long-term relationships, stable happiness, as well as sleep, appetite, and overall digestive health. In fact, a large majority of the serotonin in the body is actually stored in the intestines. Many antidepressants have serotonin in them so that they can regulate the difficult moods of people dealing with anxiety and depression. Because serotonin is more about long-term reward, children can struggle with it. If children have dangerously low levels of serotonin, they might have poor regulation and trouble controlling themselves. Thus, it is essential to make sure that your child develops proper serotonin levels. When it comes to regulating the body in many different ways, serotonin is essential.

Norepinephrine

Norepinephrine, also known as noradrenaline, or simply adrenaline, is a key part of your brain and body's stress response. When you encounter a stressful situation, norepinephrine is the chemical that is pulsating through your brain. It raises your vitals and gives you excess energy so that you can respond with maximum efficiency in a stressful scenario. In tense situations, anxiety and raised vitals are a good thing—they can help you escape from physical dangers or think clearly in a crisis—but when you have too much, they can persist and cause anxiety disorders. Many children, especially those with ADHD, can develop anxiety disorders, often during transitional or developmental periods such as early adolescence, so it's important that they keep their levels of norepinephrine in check and don't risk getting stuck in a prolonged stress response.

Glutamate

Glutamate is one of the most essential brain chemicals, important for almost all of the brain's main functions. Glutamate affects some of the most integral cognitive functions, such as memory and learning. As a result, it is one of the building blocks of early childhood development. Your child will need a significant amount of glutamate to ensure that they are storing memories properly so they turn into learning experiences. When children are young, their brains are like sponges. They are soaking up information at an alarming rate. This is why children can learn languages and instruments at a much faster rate than adults. Everything is new to them, so when a second language or a musical instrument is introduced into their world, they incorporate it into their foundational thinking. You are literally making these things a part of your child's base worldview when you are providing them with these services and it is all thanks to glutamate. Thus, your child should have a healthy amount of glutamate in their system in order to be able to successfully do what children do best, *learn*.

Hormones

The other major component of the brain that plays a huge factor in both development and mental health are hormones. Brain hormones are integral to the way the brain functions. As your child develops, their hormone balances will fundamentally shift, stimulating things like growth, mental development, and even huge transitions like puberty. Hormones can also help them regulate their mental health, feel things for others, and accomplish any number of mental tasks. They can also have a relationship to gender and sex, although these relationships are somewhat more complicated than what is conventionally taught. In this section, we will talk about hormones, what they are, and how they affect your child's brain development.

Difference Between Hormones and Neurotransmitters

People often confuse hormones for neurotransmitters, but they are actually quite different. Neurotransmitters, though they can have a relationship to the rest of the body, are fundamentally part of the brain. Hormones, on the other hand, have a relationship to the entire body, being transmitted through the bloodstream and into various parts of the body. Hormones and neurotransmitters are also part of fundamentally different systems within the body. Neurotransmitters are part of the nervous system, which relate to the spinal cord and nerve endings throughout the body, whereas hormones are a part of the endocrine system, which consists of glands such as the pituitary gland, the thyroid, and the ovaries/testicles. Thus, hormones have more to do with the functions of the endocrine system, such as sleep, mood, blood pressure, physical growth, and metabolism. Just like how people can have neurotransmitter imbalances, which can lead to mental and even physical health problems, so too can people have hormonal imbalances, which can lead to serious problems like metabolic dysfunction, insomnia, digestive issues, and much more. As you can see, hormones and neurotransmitters are kind of like two sides of the same coin, serving contrasting functions and creating harmony within the body.

Important Hormones

All hormones in the body are important, but there are a few that are the most common and produce some of the most integral functions. Ideally, everyone should have a good balance of all the hormones. (Contrary to popular belief, males have healthy doses of estrogen and females healthy doses of testosterone, which all fluctuate throughout life and even throughout the day). These hormones can have a massive effect on the way that you live your life. For children, it can affect the way they grow, feel about themselves, and deal with problems such as ADHD. In this section, we will look at some of the most central hormones within the body and how they work.

- Insulin

    o Insulin is one of the body's main hormones, which exists in the pancreas. It is responsible mainly for fat storage and metabolic regulation. You have probably heard of insulin in relation to the condition of diabetes. Diabetics have a problem with their pancreas and thus can't process sugars in the same way that others can. Thus, they have to take insulin supplements in order to be able to metabolize properly. If your insulin levels are off, you might have problems with your metabolism, even if you aren't diabetic. For example, high levels of insulin can lead to hypoglycemia, which can cause severe irritability when hungry. A well-regulated level of insulin is integral for a healthy body and metabolism.

- Melatonin

  - Also known as the "sleep hormone," melatonin is responsible for regulating your energy levels and sleepiness levels. Melatonin is responsible for your internal clock that dictates when you fall asleep and wake up. It's the reason you get naturally tired at the same time each night and will wake up, even without an alarm, in the mornings. But like insulin, melatonin can become deregulated. If you have too much, it can result in types of narcolepsy, where you constantly feel the urge to fall asleep. Too little, and you might suffer from insomnia. For children, sleep is essential for growth and development, so it is essential that they have properly-regulated melatonin so that they can have proper sleep and thus better development.

- Cortisol

  - Cortisol is the stress hormone. It is the hormonal equivalent to norepinephrine, regulating and promoting your body's stress response. If you don't have enough cortisol,

44

you will not feel a sense of danger. You will be underwhelmed at stressful situations and thus de-incentivised to work hard to escape from danger. Thankfully, because of natural selection, most people have a good amount of cortisol helping to keep us from danger. But like norepinephrine, this hormone can be dangerous in too high quantities. If you have chronically high cortisol, then you might get stuck in a constant stress loop, perceiving danger where there is none and having difficulty relaxing or calming yourself down. When children experience chronically high cortisol, they are in danger of developing an anxiety disorder or an insecure attachment style, which can cause emotional stuntedness as an adult.

- Estrogen
  - Often known as the "female hormone," estrogen is actually found in everybody, though female-born people tend to have higher levels of estrogen than male-born people. But despite this, having too high or too low estrogen is dangerous for everybody. Chronically high estrogen can lead to depression and infertility, while chronically low estrogen can lead to loss of bone density and cardiovascular disease.

This is why menopausal women who lose estrogen very quickly tend to break bones easily. But even as a child, everyone needs their estrogen levels in line, especially approaching the onset of puberty.

- Testosterone

  ○ Often known as the "male hormone," testosterone is, again, found in everybody, though it is somewhat more prevalent in male-born bodies. Like estrogen, testosterone also affects bone density, resulting in more brittle bones if testosterone levels are lower. Another part of the body majorly affected by testosterone is muscle mass. Many bodybuilders will take testosterone supplements to help grow their muscle mass. But even in children, regulated testosterone levels are necessary for normal and healthy development.

ADHD Vs Non-ADHD Brain

So how do all these elements interact with ADHD? What do we talk about when we talk about child and developmental ADHD anyways? Well, throughout the last section, we frequently mentioned some of the things that can go wrong with all the various brain parts, neurotransmitters, and hormones that are present in the brain. For your child to develop in a healthy way, they will need many of these things to be regulated. Obviously no one is perfect, and everyone will have some sort of chemical or hormonal imbalance at some point throughout their life. But children with ADHD have a different experience of development than children without. In this section, we will talk about some of the aspects of the brain that are particularly affected by ADHD and vice versa, enlightening you about how your child's brain might be developing slightly differently from others'.

Structural Development

One of the main differences between brain development in those with ADHD and those without is structural development. The brains of those with ADHD take a bit longer than others to develop. As such, they might resemble the brain parts of a younger child. This of course doesn't mean that your child is 'slow' or dumb, it merely means that they struggle more than others with very specific functions. The parts of the brain that the ADHD child particularly struggles with are the caudate nucleus (decision making), the putamen (learning and memory), the hippocampus (working memory), the amygdala (emotional control), the nucleus accumbens (mood and pleasure), and of course, the cerebral cortex or prefrontal cortex (self-regulation). As you can see, many of the functions of these brain components are qualities that people with ADHD tend to struggle with. In the case of children's development, we can physically see how these parts of the brain are actually smaller. Thus, if you find your child struggling with something like learning or emotional control, you can remind yourself that they have a physically smaller amygdala or putamen than other children their age and try to build understanding around that. With the right exercises, however, your children can start to build these skills, working around their different brains and helping to gain some of these functions through hard work.

Networking

There is a popular phrase in neuroscience known as "neurons that fire together wire together." This saying is illustrating the power of connections made within the brain. The brain is made of millions of cells called neurons. These neurons fire signals at one another which form the basis of thoughts. When certain neurons connect often, meaning you are frequently thinking a certain thought, this means that they are "firing together." And as the saying goes, they are incentivised to "wire together," or form a connection. This is how habits form, as well as memories, ideas, and frameworks about the world. All of learning and forming memories is creating connections between your neurons and thus this firing and wiring function is a fundamental part of a developing brain.

However, children with ADHD tend to struggle with this function. Their brains actually take physically longer to form these fundamental connections or pathways through the brain. So, while it might take a non-ADHD child five 'fires' to 'wire,' it might take a child with ADHD ten or even twenty. This manifests in the real world through ADHD children taking longer to learn things or form habits. A non-ADHD child might be able to deeply internalize a math concept with five practices, while it might take ten or twenty tries to get the child with ADHD to learn the same thing. This is a big reason why common accommodations for those with ADHD are simply more time to complete homework and more one-on-one help to complete assignments. If they are simply given more time, they can often learn just as effectively as someone without ADHD, simply needing those extra 'fires' in order to create the essential 'wires' in their brains. Again, this simple ADHD quality can all be broken down into neuroscience!

Neurotransmitters

Back in the last section, we talked a lot about neurotransmitters and their functions. In relation to neuron connections, we can see how important these transmitters are in forming essential connections between neurons and creating learned behavior and memories. As you can probably infer, most children with ADHD have a deficiency in certain essential neurotransmitters. When children with ADHD experience deficiency in certain neurotransmitters, it can mean that they again struggle to make and keep connections within their brain. Many ADHD medications include supplements of these essential neurotransmitters, helping the child with ADHD to improve their neuron connections and thus learn better. Brain training such as cognitive behavioral therapy (or CBT) can also help to naturally boost neurotransmitters. Some psychologists have found that tapping into a child's interests (and thus boosting neurotransmitters like dopamine and serotonin) can help to improve the flow of neurotransmitters. When it comes to ADHD, brain chemistry is incredibly important.

The Brain-Body Connection

But it's not just the brain that is affected and affects ADHD. The body has an important role to play in the world of mental health. More and more throughout the last few years, scientists have been researching ways in which the body interacts with mental health, especially mental health issues. They have started promoting more holistic ways to treat mental health, such as through diet and exercise, helping people to target areas of the body that might improve their mental health. When it comes to ADHD, the body can play a significant factor in both causing, affecting, and curing ADHD. Thus, focusing solely on the mind creates a limited view of your child's condition and might cause them to miss out on treatments that might benefit them. Understanding how the body and mind connect with one another can help you to understand your child's ADHD more thoroughly and create a stronger connection between their mind and body. In this section, we will talk about how the mind and body are connected in relation to ADHD.

ADHD and the Body

So what is the relationship between ADHD and the body? It's no secret that a healthy body makes for a healthy mind, but what exactly are the components of a healthy body and how do they specifically contribute to the health of the mind? Many ADHD experts have studied how various conditions of the body can actually have a massive effect on the way that children with ADHD function. In this section, we will talk about the ways in which physical health can impact ADHD. There are four main components that we will talk about. First, we will discuss the role of nutrition in the ADHD brain of a child. Then, we will talk about physical activity and how that can improve ADHD symptoms in children. After that, we will talk about some up-and-coming research in gut health and how that can have a strong connection with brain chemistry and neurotransmitters. Finally, we will talk about the nervous system and the role it has to play in children's ADHD development. By the end of this section, you should have a good idea of how the body can greatly affect ADHD symptoms and recovery.

Nutrition

We all know that eating healthy is good for you, but why exactly? What do fruits and vegetables do to the body that makes us so healthy? Well, there are many ways in which the foods we eat affect our overall health, as well as our mental health. For ADHD in particular, there might be some foods you want to encourage or avoid to help mitigate symptoms and improve cognitive function. Here, we will give you a list of foods that you should avoid and encourage to improve cognition in ADHD children.

Foods to Avoid

When it comes to diets, it's best to encourage good foods, rather than discourage 'bad' foods. This is for several reasons. For one, banning foods can actually create a forbidden fruit narrative, making children crave them more. And second of all, there are no 'bad' foods that you should never eat under any circumstances, only foods that you shouldn't eat as often. That being said, if you have a child with ADHD, there are some foods you should generally avoid giving them. Here is a general list of some of the categories you might want to avoid giving to children with ADHD.

- Caffeine
    - The most obvious thing you should avoid with ADHD children is caffeine. Children in general shouldn't have caffeine, since it is considered to be a highly stimulating drug, but ADHD children especially shouldn't have it, particularly children who are more on the hyperactive side, for obvious reasons. Caffeine can also cause anxiety, which ADHD children are prone to, so you should avoid it at all costs. You might think keeping them away from coffee and tea is enough, but many 'kid-friendly' foods and drinks also contain caffeine. Chocolate, especially dark chocolate, as well as many sodas like Coke and Pepsi all contain caffeine, so if your child has ADHD, you might have to limit their consumption of these things.

- Sugar
    - Another stimulating substance is of course sugar. Sugar is similar to caffeine in the sense that it gives you a short but intense burst of energy that then dissipates very quickly. Children with ADHD might struggle more with these intense rushes and crashes, especially considering attention and energy inconsistency is a trademark of ADHD, and so sugar can often exacerbate that. Obviously, sugar is in a lot of

things, so there is no avoiding it completely. However, if you can limit your child's sugar intake in general, especially in large quantities at once, you can help to avoid some of the energy rushes and crashes that come along with it.

- Mercury-rich foods

  o Recently, a lot more medical studies have been done about the harmful effects of mercury on the mind and body, especially in the long-term. It is a very difficult substance to digest and thus can cause a whole host of issues. It is particularly harmful to the brain, where it builds up and causes hyperactivity. Most fish contain some levels of mercury, and so you should be careful with the amount of fish your child with ADHD eats. Occasional fish is fine, but perhaps not every single day. Be wary of the possible long-term implications of feeding your child too much mercury-rich foods.

- Foods they have sensitivities to

  o Certain symptoms of ADHD, such as anxiety and brain fog, can be greatly exacerbated by exposure to allergens. If your child has any allergies or food sensitivities, it is imperative that you avoid them at all costs with no exceptions. They might be contributing to your child's ADHD symptoms and so you should leave them off as much as you can. Even something as innocuous-seeming as lactose intolerance can be contributing, so make sure your child stays away from dairy at all costs in this case. If you aren't sure if your child has sensitivities, it is a good idea to get them allergy tested with your doctor to make sure they aren't consuming anything that might be harmful to them and exacerbating their ADHD.

Foods to Encourage

But it's not all about restriction! There are of course still many things your child can and should be eating to help with their ADHD. One of the most common issues that can be caused by and also contribute to ADHD, is vitamin deficiencies. There are many vitamins within the body that need to be maintained and can cause devastating consequences if they aren't. If you suspect that your child might have vitamin deficiencies, put them on a good multivitamin to get their nutrients up and then change their diet to include the following list of nutrients. After a while, you can take them off the multivitamin so that they can get all their nutrients naturally. You should also make sure your child is getting enough roughage to make sure they maintain a healthy digestive system. Here, we will look at some of the most essential vitamins and the foods that contain them for your child to maintain a healthy diet with ADHD.

- Protein
  - To maintain consistent and high energy levels, as well as build muscle, you should make sure that your child has a diet rich in protein. Traditionally, people tend to think of red meat, things like steaks and burgers to be the only sources of protein, but with more awareness around plant-based eating, people are opening up to more diverse sources of protein. Foods like nuts, soy, beans, eggs, and of course, fish and poultry, are some of the best sources of protein for your child. Try serving them more peanut butter for snacks to give them a little protein boost throughout the day.

- Omega-3 fatty acids
  - Also known as the "brain vitamin," Omega-3 fatty acids are a very important vitamin for cognitive function. Since ADHD greatly affects cognitive abilities and development, you want to make sure that your child has as much of it as possible. Some of the highest sources of Omega-3 are in fish, especially tuna and salmon. Since these can contain harmful mercury levels, you could consider feeding

your child fish oil or Omega-3 supplements instead to avoid mercury.

- B vitamins
  - Vitamin B-6 and B-12 are some of the most important aspects of a mental health diet. These both greatly affect your mood and many studies have shown that people with anxiety tend to have chronically low vitamin B-12. Meat and dairy are the best sources of B12, whereas leafy greens are an excellent source of B-6.

- Fruits and vegetables
  - You can never get enough of the old standby — fresh fruits and vegetables are incredibly important to the maintenance of a healthy diet. Not only do they contain many of some of the most essential nutrients, but they also contain roughage and hydration, meaning that your child is getting more out of them than they would a multivitamin. Some studies suggest that the ratio of fresh fruits and vegetables to all other foods should be 50%, meaning that for every calorie your child eats in meat, carbs, or anything else, they should have a calorie from fruits or vegetables. This might sound like a lot, but it is absolutely worth it for the physical and mental health of your child.

Activity

Diet isn't the only thing that matters when it comes to improving your child's health. Physical activity is very important to the mind and body. And people aren't getting enough of it. Due to more car-centric and screen-centric lifestyles, more children and teens are staying inside and exercising less. It is estimated that as much as 80% of teenagers don't meet the requirements for physical activity laid out by WHO (*Physical Activity*, 2022). To get a sense of how much physical activity your child should be getting, children ages 5–17 are recommended 60 minutes of physical activity a day and to limit the amount of time they are completely sedentary. If that sounds like a lot, then it is likely your child is not receiving the amount of physical activity they need.

For kids with ADHD, this is an even more important requirement. As we have talked about throughout this book, children with ADHD have a lot of excess energy. This excess energy can be channeled into physical activity, such as sports, dance, or other such activities. These can both improve your child's physical health, as well as give them a focus for some of their energy. You might find that if you improve your child's physical activity levels, they fidget and misbehave less because they are using up their excess energy for a more constructive purpose. And finally, simply improving overall health will improve your child's mental health. Even if they aren't a particularly hyperactive or over energetic kid, they will still benefit immensely from having more physical activity in their life.

Gut Health

We might not like to think of our intestines. It doesn't seem like they perform any specific function that is too important. We tend to think of the stomach as doing all the heavy lifting within the digestive system, but that actually isn't true. In fact, our guts do almost all of the nutrient absorption within our bodies. This means that all those good vitamins you want your kids to be eating won't actually get absorbed unless their gut is functioning properly. Disastrous things happen when the gut malfunctions. Celiac's disease, a genetic autoimmune disorder, prevents the intestinal lining from absorbing nutrients which can lead to chronic and even dangerous malnourishment and vitamin deficiencies. Thus, it is incredibly important to have your gut health in order. Eating plenty of fiber, drinking lots of water, and even introducing fermented foods such as kombucha, kimchi, and yogurt into your child's diet can greatly improve their gut health. As we said back in the section on neurotransmitters, much of the body's serotonin is created in the cits and thus you should make sure they are taken care of as much as possible for the sake of your child's mental health.

Health Issues and ADHD

There are actually several underlying health conditions that can cause or affect ADHD. If your child has ADHD, there is a chance that it might actually be caused by an underlying health or hormonal problem that has gone undiagnosed. Of course, there are many complex factors that contribute to ADHD and your child does not necessarily have another health condition if they have ADHD, but you should look into it anyways. Some health conditions associated with ADHD are fetal alcohol syndrome, vitamin deficiencies, Celiac's disease.

CHAPTER 3:

WHAT CAN I DO AS A PARENT

As the parent of a child with ADHD, it can seem really overwhelming and at times you can start to feel helpless. Your child might be in states that you simply cannot shake them out of, meaning that you are left wondering what exactly you are supposed to be doing to help the situation. The answer is a two-pronged approach. First of all, you need to let go of the idea that you have 100% control over your child. You have control over their environment and over the kind of family life they have, but that is where your control ends. Their own unique brain chemistry and the world outside your home have a powerful effect on your child that you simply cannot control and accepting that is part of being a parent. Second of all, you can learn strategies for how to deal with your child's ADHD, especially their outbursts or more distressing symptoms, in order to feel less helpless. The good news is that you don't *have* to be helpless. You can do so many things to help your child, especially with the right education, and so there is no need to feel helpless.

In this chapter, we will show you all the important aspects of creating an environment in which your child feels safe, supported, and at the same times structured and disciplined. First, we will discuss how to tailor-fit this environment and approach your child specifically. There is no way to dictate a "one-size-fits-all" approach to ADHD parenting. The specific symptoms and personality of your child are integral to your success as an ADHD parent. Next, we will talk about strategies for creating that environment, what kinds of things you need and how you should implement it for your child. And lastly, we will discuss the importance of modeling the behaviors you want to encourage in your child, positioning yourself as the ultimate role model for them. By the end of this chapter, you should start to be able to waive some of those intense feelings of helplessness that you might have had upon your child's initial diagnosis and start working towards more tangible improvements!

No "One-Size-Fits-All"

If you've ever given out t-shirts at a large event, you have likely learned that "one-size fits-all" tends to be a bit of a lie. In practice, one size generally doesn't fit all, or at least fits very differently on all who try it. Different shirts will look completely different on different body types, creating just as much difference as if you had given everyone a range of sizes in the first place. Ideally, everyone would get to pick their size and have a shirt that fits them. Even more ideally, everyone would get to go to a tailor and have their shirt fitted to their body's exact unique proportions. But in a world based on maximum efficiency, we tend to have one-size-fits-all solutions to many of life's problems, which can lead to a whole host of complications. The medical system, the education system, and many more mass-scale systems are based on huge one-size-fits-all approaches like standardized testing and minimum requirements. On this massive scale, that's just the way things have to be so that they work efficiently.

But your home doesn't work like that. You and your child have a special relationship that could never be dictated by rules or standards. You wouldn't give your child a present based on the statistical most popular toy amongst their age group, you would give them a present based on what you know of their interests. You wouldn't treat two of your children exactly the same, knowing that each has unique areas of interest and needs that make them into a special person. So even outside of ADHD, you are not treating your child with a standardized approach. But when it comes to something like ADHD, which you likely have absolutely no experience with, you probably find yourself reaching for more standardized approaches, purely out of confusion. You might find yourself searching "how to treat your ADHD child," or things of the like. But what is most important to realize is that they are still your child. They still have all the unique characteristics that you love about them and that make them unique. Thus, their ADHD will also have unique qualities that will create unique needs. When you are supporting them as a parent, you thus need to be able to tailor their treatment to the way they are. In this chapter, we will talk about the ways in which you can get to know your child a little better through the lens of ADHD and thus work towards a completely customized experience.

Observing Their Habits

Before you can assess what your child might need, you need to figure out what they're actual experience of ADHD is. Chances are, your child has more symptoms than just the initial ones that led you to get them tested. There are hundreds of minor or less common ADHD symptoms that your child might be experiencing without you realizing it. Before you observe your child, you need to make sure to read every list you can find of ADHD symptoms and genuinely reflect on whether you think your child is exhibiting that sign. Then, you need to write down all that you think might apply. Following this, you need to put that list into action. Choose a day when your child is at home, or sit-in in their school classroom and observe what they do in a day. Try not to make them feel like they're being watched. You don't need to be staring at them the entire time, just make notes of things like what they eat, how long they watch TV for, whether or not they procrastinate their homework, whether they seem frustrated or cranky, how easily they wake up in the morning or go to bed at night. Making note of these things can help you get a sense of how ADHD is contributing to your child's day and how you might be able to help them through it going forward. These notes will give you a framework for what you actually want to improve in your child's life and what symptoms of ADHD you think they need support for.

Working With Their Personality and Interests

As we said in the last chapter, finding a person with ADHD's unique points of interest can really help them to break out of some of the negative cycles they find themselves in. Similarly, just knowing what your child is particularly interested in can help you focus on their strengths while helping to support some of their weaknesses. There are two sides to this portion, or two types of interests that you should be paying attention to, either their material interests, such as the kinds of books, movies, or subjects they enjoy learning about, and their talents, such as their listening skills, reading level, or verbal skills. Highlighting both of these types of strengths can not only help you to build your child's self-esteem, but also hijack the things they are good at to help them succeed in life. Here, we will talk about these two types of interests/talents and how you can use them to your and your child's advantage in parenting them through your ADHD.

Material Interests

The first kind of interest is the subjects your child likes. Maybe it's a video game or comic book series they can't get enough of. Maybe it's dinosaurs or outer space and they love nothing more than going to the museum and learning about those subjects. Maybe it's a sport that they get lost in whenever they play, or their after school guitar lesson. Whatever it is, it's highly likely that your child has some sort of interest that they are passionate about. Even if they suffer from severe ADHD, it's likely that they still have something that can hold their interest and get them excited about learning. As a parent, it's really important to recognize this, both to acknowledge your child's admirable curiosity, but also to have a jumping off point for when you are trying to help them with other aspects of life. For example, your child might really struggle with reading. Try as you might, they just don't seem to be able to hold interest for longer than a page. One strategy would be to buy them a book about something they're really passionate about. They might not be too incentivized to read a novel for school, but if they have a passion for space travel and you buy them an encyclopedia of stars and planets, they might be more incentivized to keep reading because they enjoy the material. Finding ways to incorporate your child's special interests into something that they enjoy can help to hold their attention a little longer than they may have otherwise.

Strengths

Besides their personal interests, your child also has certain things they're good at. Maybe they have a mature vocal cadence and are good at talking to adults. Maybe they are an amazing artist when they put their mind to it. Maybe they are very naturally curious and will always try a new food or movie if it is offered to them. These strengths are more personality-based rather than interest-based, but you can still use them to your advantage when you are trying to find accommodations for them. For example, if your child really has a hard time writing, can't seem to string a sentence together with a pencil, but are very articulate and motor mouthed when they talk, you could try using a speech-to-text program to translate your child's musings into writing, which you can then go over with them and edit. This can help them feel more accomplished, like they actually wrote something, and actually materially improve their ability to produce schoolwork. On the flipside, you might have a child who is incredibly withdrawn and can barely make eye contact with others, but can write very well. You might encourage them to read a speech they wrote in front of the class to practice being vocally vulnerable, but while still playing to their writing strength. Accommodations that not just address the major symptoms of ADHD, but also play to your child's specific strengths can have a massive impact on the way they overcome their ADHD symptoms.

Asking How They Feel

And finally, one of the best things you can do to get to know your child and their experience of ADHD better is to simply ask them yourself. Opening lines of communication between the two of you is excellent for creating a collaborative process towards recovery. After all, if you don't have the cooperation of your child during their ADHD treatment, you will have a much harder time getting them the help they need and making sure it sticks. As the old joke goes: "It only takes one psychiatrist to screw in a lightbulb, but the lightbulb has to want to change." If you include your child in your curation of their ADHD recovery methods, they will both be more on board with their treatments and gain a stronger sense of autonomy.

Some ways to include your child would be to ask them specific questions. For example, you could ask them what things frustrate them the most throughout their day. Is it getting ready in the morning? Finding time to do homework? Following instructions at school? You might find that the thing they pinpoint isn't the same thing that you would have thought. If they are masking well, they might even be succeeding at these things, but are experiencing emotional distress while doing so. Or, you could ask them what they would like to do better in life. It might be reading, learning new things, or making friends. If you connect with their wants, you will be able to more easily work towards a clear incentive and create a more solid grasp on their goals. If you make the effort to have a serious talk with your child, including them in the objectives of their ADHD treatment, then you will be able to create a more collaborative tailor-made treatment for them.

Creating Their Environment

Once you have really pinned down the things that you need to do to help your child and the way that they personally need to be accommodated, you can start making tangible changes in your own life that will start to create an environment that is more conducive to your child's ADHD. Of course, your tailor-made approach will dictate the areas and the methods you use to curate their environment, but there are still some general approaches you should take. These general tips will help you to discover and maintain your approach. From there, you can customize them to your unique child. Here, we will offer you some important tips for how to create a solid environment for your ADHD child.

Tip #1: Be Consistent

In all parenting, consistency is important. You want to make sure that you maintain consistent reward and punishment systems, create steady rules, and react similarly to similar situations so that your child can feel stable in their relationship to you and always knows where they stand. However, for an ADHD child, consistency is even more important. Children with ADHD lack structure and consistency in their own minds and so the outside world has to be twice as consistent in order to help them cope. Now, consistency doesn't have to mean boring. You might think that a consistent existence for your child means that they have to eat the same thing every day or do the same activities. But this is not the case. People with ADHD need stimulation as much as the next person, and in some cases, especially those who are consistently understimulated, need more. The trick is finding stability within variety. Consistency simply means consistent levels of stimuli, no big surprises, clear scheduling, and the same level of emotional support. So, your child might love trying lots of interesting new foods, but they always eat at the same time every day. Or, you have a family movie night every Friday, but you always make a point to watch

70

something none of you have seen before. Making sure that your child knows the level of stimulation they are getting every day and week is essential to ensuring that they can emotionally regulate themselves more easily, given that they have practice in that area.

Tip #2: Give Options

In Chapter 1, we talked about some of the major differences between adults with ADHD and children. While adults carry more responsibility, they also benefit from being able to curate their own schedules and thus have a more intuitive approach to accommodating their ADHD. Children, on the other hand, are almost always at the mercy of schedules made for them by adults, whether they are at school or home. Thus, many children, especially those with ADHD, feel powerless and cannot practice intuitive approaches. If your child suddenly feels a burst of productivity during their scheduled nap time, they won't be able to follow that instinct. Likewise, they might feel extra tired one day after school and not be in the right headspace to do their homework right away, but are beholden to it because of their scheduled homework time. If you give your children options, however, in what they can do, you allow them to have more malleability in their schedules and start to practice the adult skill of intuitive accommodations.

So what do these options look like? You might be thinking: *"That won't work – If I ask my child whether they want to do their homework or watch TV, they're obviously going to pick the latter!"* While that might be true, there are many ways you can practice optional scheduling without making such a clear dichotomy. The trick is to follow two principles: Variety of activity and rearrangement. Here, we will talk about the differences between these two approaches and how you can implement them into your child's life.

Choice of Activity

The first principle, activity options, involves giving your child a range of options within the scheduled time. So, say you have a few blocks of time in the evening, one for homework, one for downtime, and one for family time. For each of these blocks, you can offer a variety. For downtime, you could offer a few different options, not just TV, say drawing, listening to music, or going for a walk. These three low-impact activities are relaxing in the same way as watching TV, but still involve something mildly stimulating so as to still be active. This variety of options can also allow your child to choose based on their mood what *kind* of downtime they want. Do they want creative expression (drawing), creative consumption (listening to music), or light physical activity (walking)? This variety of options not only allows your child more autonomy in going with their feelings in the moment, but also encourages them to think about downtime beyond just sitting on the couch.

Rearrangement

Have you ever woken up one morning and felt like getting right to work? But then woke up the next morning and felt like all you want to do is drink your coffee and read the paper for an hour? Or another morning where you felt you just had to write in your journal or jot down some short story ideas? Everyone feels differently at fixed points between each day. Some evenings are spent out partying with friends while others are spent in front of the TV with a loved one. Likewise, your child likely wakes up or comes home from school in different moods every day. Maybe one day they didn't get much sleep and wake up cranky to the point where you can barely get them ready and out the door, much less have a productive and relaxing morning. Maybe one day they studied something really interesting at school and your child comes home excited to do their homework. Whatever the circumstances, you need to account for the fact that your child is not going to be in the same mood each day. Thus, you can use those blocks we talked about in the last section, but make them re-arrangeable. So, for example, say you schedule one hour for homework, downtime, and family time. Your child can then choose which they would like to do first. Maybe one day they feel like doing their homework first, then having some downtime, but another day they really feel like they need a break before they can do homework and thus take their downtime first. This can really help your child grow their autonomy and make sure they are using their energy wisely. If you help them make these decisions intuitively, they will be able to make these decisions into adulthood as well.

Tip #3: Be Their Advocate

It's an unfortunate reality, but not everyone is going to understand ADHD as well as you do. Not every single person in your child's life is going to have read extensive literature on ADHD and put in the work to understand all its nuances. It would be great if that were the case, but we don't live in a perfect world. Thus, you are likely going to encounter another adult, perhaps a dance teacher, a little league coach, or even a friend's parent, who becomes frustrated with your child because they simply do not understand their condition. This can be very painful for you to watch because you know how difficult a time your child has with some of these everyday tasks. But on the other hand, you also know what it's like to be frustrated with some of your child's behavior. In these situations, you need to be that intermediary between your child and that other adult. Use your understanding of both sides to explain to each where the other is coming from. Express to that other adult your child's condition and the specific symptoms they experience and explain that it isn't their fault. You can even share some tips for managing these symptoms that you have found work for yourself. For your child, remind them regularly that not everyone understands what they are going through and help them to gain the vocabulary and knowledge to explain their condition to others even when you are not around. Being your child's advocate, as well as teaching them to advocate for themselves, will help them to navigate the world outside of your home, turning all their environments into supportive ones.

Modeling Healthy Habits Yourself

In Stephen Sondheim's classic musical *Into the Woods*, famously about relationships between parents and children, the theme of the opening number states: "Children may not obey, but children will listen." This piece of wisdom will likely ring true to any parent. Your child might not do what you tell them to do, but they will absorb everything you say and do and oftentimes mimic it. It's probably why you have sometimes found your child saying oddly adult-sounding phrases, parroting your exact language, or when you find them not listening to your advice to avoid something they've seen you do. If you want to maintain credibility, but also provide a good role model for your child, you need to model the kind of behavior you want them to build into their life. In the next chapter, we will expand on this idea of modeling good behavior as a parent, discussing the role of your own behaviors in your child's ADHD recovery.

CHAPTER 4:

PUT ON YOUR
OXYGEN MASK FIRST

When you are in an airplane, the oxygen masks clearly state that you must put on your own oxygen mask before you help someone else with theirs, even if they are a child. This instruction might be counter-intuitive, especially for the more empathetic among us. However, it is actually very good and practical advice.

When you put on your own oxygen mask, you ensure that you are able to breathe while you help the next person. Otherwise, you might pass out while helping them and then no one gets their mask on. While this is true in a literal sense, there is also a metaphorical truth to it. If you aren't healthy or able, you cannot help others. Children need parents who are attentive, yes, but also parents who are healthy enough themselves to be able to give them the help they need. If you are not getting enough sleep, eating properly, and taking enough time for your mental health, then you are not going to be parenting your child to the fullest extent of your abilities. This is especially true if you have a child with special needs like ADHD, requiring you to go that extra mile more than other parents. In other words, you need to be making sure you are healthy before you can try to help your child be healthier.

In this chapter, we will turn the conversation towards you and give you some important advice on how to manage your own mental health while parenting an ADHD child. First, we will talk about the possible issues that can arise if you have an unhealthy lifestyle as a parent, illustrating the effect that has on a child, especially one with ADHD. Then, we will talk about an important distinction in mental healthcare between self-care and healthy habits, helping you to meet all sides of your needs. And finally, we will talk about how you can work towards a healthy balance of meeting your own needs and your child's needs. After finishing this chapter, you should have a good sense of your own role to play in your child's ADHD recovery and how you can make sure to keep yourself safe and healthy throughout the process.

The Dangers of an Unhealthy Parent

No one is perfectly healthy. Who among us has never skipped their daily veggies or neglected to get our 10,000 steps? Who has never engaged in a little extra drinking at a party or stayed out all night in the cold? Humans engage in unhealthy behavior all the time and, for the most part, if done in moderation, it's fairly harmless. However, the real harm begins when it becomes chronic. Skipping the gym a few days in a row is much better than never making any time for physical exercise in your life. Having a fast food meal once in a while is much different from it being a staple in your diet. Staying up all night once a year is much better than consistently getting less than six hours every night. The more chronic the unhealthy behavior, the more it is going to take its toll on your mind and body. From there, it will greatly affect your mood and your energy levels. And as you know from being a long-time parent, these things are essential to creating a strong relationship with your children. Getting insufficient sleep means you are less attentive to them throughout the day. Having an unhealthy diet or nonexistent exercise regime means you won't be fit enough to run around with them at the park. Neglecting your personal issues means you will have backed up resentment and frustrations that will seep into your dealings with them. Even though it might not seem like it, having an unhealthy lifestyle can actually be indirectly harmful to your children. This is not to shame anyone's parenting, but to make you see how important taking care of yourself is both for your happiness and your child's. In this section, we will discuss the different aspects of health and how they might affect your child's health.

General Health and Wellness

In terms of general physical health, it might not seem like that will greatly affect your parenting, but it actually does. There are a few ways in which your general health is incredibly important to who you are as a parent. First of all, the way that you eat and exercise has a role in your child's habits. According to a study by Duke Medicine, children whose parents modeled healthy eating and exercise habits were less likely to be obese (*Parenting and Home Environment Influence Children's Exercise and Eating Habits*, n.d.) with the greater influence being in nutrition. Since we talked back in Chapter 2 about how important physical health and nutrition are in ADHD recovery, the health of the parent is significant in how children overcome ADHD. The other way in which your physical health impacts your child and their ADHD recovery is through your ability to be present. A healthier diet and a consistent exercise regime have been time and again linked to higher cognitive function, better emotional stability, and higher alertness. If you are making sure that your brain and body are fed properly, you are making sure that your child has a caregiver who is at the top of their game and ready to deal with whatever life throws at them. And it's not just diet and exercise, it's sleep too! More and more recent research on chronic sleep deprivation (getting less than the recommended 6-8 hours) has been measuring its negative impact on the mind and body. Failing to get proper sleep, eat healthy, and exercise can thus very negatively affect your and your child's health, possibly even hindering their ADHD recovery.

Mental Health Issues

Just like the universal tendency to skip out on healthy things once in a while, we all have our own issues. No one has gone through life without experiencing some level of trauma or regret, nor is anyone's life perfect. These things can absolutely get in the way of your parenting. You probably remember a time when you felt like your parents were taking out their own issues on you, perhaps by punishing you when you didn't really deserve it or lacking the patience to listen to your problems. But have no fear if you have mental health issues: The distinction isn't in our level of issues, it's in how you deal with them. If you don't seek out help for your mental health, be that from a therapist, friend, or partner, then you run the very real risk of taking them out on your children and potentially passing those issues onto them.

Another difficult situation that can occur with particularly mentally ill parents is a process called parentification, wherein parents rely on their children for psychological support, forcing the child to act as an emotional caregiver. While it is good to rely on loved ones for support, you should never rely on a child. They do not have the emotional tools to help you and asking them to do so will only burden them with the guilt that they can't help you. If you need help for your mental health, you need to make sure you get that from another adult. Children are not capable of giving you that support, instead needing you to do that for them. And for a child who is also suffering from ADHD, additional mental health issues are not welcome. When you properly manage your own mental health, you can protect your children from potentially being on the receiving end of it, and can thus focus exclusively on helping them through their own issues, as the caregiver should.

Could You Have ADHD?

One possibility to consider is whether or not you have ADHD. Many people who were born before the 21st century have gone undiagnosed. Back then, there was not the same level of awareness around mental health, especially ADHD, and so people who may have been exhibiting lots of symptoms were not flagged for the condition. If you, while reading the first half of this book, came across some symptoms that rang true to you, there is a very real possibility that you in fact have ADHD. Some studies even show that ADHD can be hereditary or at least tends to run in families, and so if your child has ADHD, there is actually a stronger likelihood that you have it as well. Finding out if you have ADHD, getting diagnosed, and seeking treatment is just as important as doing so for your child. Many older people feel as though it is too late for them, that it doesn't matter whether they get diagnosed or not, but this couldn't be further from the truth. There are many adults getting diagnosed with ADHD every single day and many of them find that it greatly improves their quality of life. It can also help your relationship with your child. Seeking treatment for your ADHD will help you take back control of your attention and be more present for your child. Plus, going through ADHD treatment together can actually help you greatly bond with your child and grow your relationship. You will be able to better understand where they are coming from and vice versa. So, if you think there is even a slight possibility that you have ADHD, it would be highly beneficial for you and your child to get testing and treatment as soon as possible.

Self-Care and Healthy Habits

Now that you understand how devastating it can be to have terribly unhealthy habits as a parent and how integral it is to develop healthy ones, you need to understand what those healthy habits are. The first thing to say right off the bat is that you never have to feel guilty for prioritizing these things. There are a lot of narratives out there that parents have to be completely selfless, but that couldn't be further from the truth. There is nothing noble about letting your health slide for the sake of your children. Keep in mind that you deserve a healthy lifestyle and that doing so will likely benefit your children as well. So, how do you achieve this healthy lifestyle? What kind of healthy habits should you engage in to help yourself achieve better mental and physical health? Well, here, we are going to talk about a two-pronged method that involves prioritizing both self-care and healthy habits. First, we will talk about the distinction between these two things and why they're both important. After that, we will talk about the 5 pillars of healthy habits to encapsulate all your basic human needs. Then, we will discuss the ins and outs of self-care, giving you some key self-care activities that you can engage in.

What's the Difference?

So why the distinction between self-care and healthy habits? Well, the distinction comes down to basics versus idiosyncrasies, or wants versus needs. Healthy habits are the more general categories everyone needs to fulfill in order to be a healthy person, whereas self-care is about feeding your individual wants and unique needs. So, eating a healthy diet would be a healthy habit, but taking time to go to a nice restaurant because that's something that brings you joy would be self-care. Both of these things are important in order to have a happy and healthy lifestyle and, most importantly, to be a good parent. It might feel like being a parent means that your life is no longer your own, that you don't have a scrap of free time. You might think you simply don't have the time, money, or energy for self-care. But this is not a healthy way to live. Many of the habits and self-care activities we will talk about next actually don't cost you that much more time and money while offering you infinite rewards. In the next two sections, we will offer you some very important tips for how to implement healthier and conscious living into your life.

Healthy Habits: Covering Your 5 Basic Needs

We all have basic needs that cover our needs in life. One of the most famous frameworks of needs-based living was laid out by Maslow in his hierarchy of needs, which laid out five basic areas of need that all humans have. This list started the conversation around separating basic needs into categories. For the purposes of this section, we have created a list of five healthy habits based around five basic needs, loosely based on Maslow's hierarchy of needs.

Basic Need #1: Nutrition

As we have talked about throughout this chapter, making sure you are eating the right foods is essential. Refer back to the section on nutrition from Chapter 2 to understand the basic foods you should be eating. Try to get your five servings of fruit and vegetables from fresh sources, eat whole grains, and drink plenty of water. Do research into things like your gender, age group, and potential health conditions to curate the ideal healthy diet for yourself. Of course, there's no shame in 'cheating' once in a while and indulging in a treat. In fact, most experts say that controlled desserts and treats can actually help make a diet more sustainable. This is not about losing weight or going on some crazy crash diet. All you need to do is implement healthier foods into your diet, not worrying about completely eliminating 'unhealthy' foods. This dietary practice will form the basis of your healthy habits. If you are feeding your body with what it needs, then it will be able to perform the rest of your essential needs properly.

Basic Need #2: Moving Your Body

Exercise is an incredibly important part of life. Our bodies are not meant to be sitting down all day, cooped up inside. We evolved to be active creatures, running and walking and dancing. Thus, living an exclusively sedentary lifestyle where you drive everywhere, never go to the gym, and don't play any sports means that you are treating your body in a way that is harmful. It might not seem like harm, because you aren't doing anything to it, but neglecting to use your muscles means that your body is not happy and not working the way it should. Exercise has also been proven to improve mood and cognitive function, so it is also important for your mental health that you engage in exercise. Again, this is not about losing weight or becoming a bodybuilder. There's no need to rush and sign up for a gym membership. The best way to exercise in a way that you know is going to be consistent is to find something that you enjoy and that fits into your lifestyle. Some people choose to start walking or cycling to work instead of driving, or join a dance or martial arts class, or even to do daily morning yoga. Whatever piques your interest, gets your body moving, and doesn't take you too far out of your way is a sustainable way for you to implement exercise into your life.

Basic Need #3: Relationships

As the famous John Donne titled his book, *No Man is an Island*, all human beings need to have relationships in order to maintain our sanity and our sense of self. Relationships are more than just offering us someone to talk to or a shoulder to cry on. They are what make us who we are. If you are not having fulfilling relationships in your life, or prioritizing the ones that you do have, you can fall into a pit of loneliness. It's no secret that maintaining friendships after you have children is really difficult, but it is still important to prioritize trying to do so. Another important aspect of your relationship needs is to have a variety of relationships. You have your children, and possibly a spouse, but you should also have strong friendships, professional connections, and acquaintances in your community. The latter is often overlooked, but actually one of the most important things to have. Feeling like you are a strong member of a community is an important necessity in life. So when you are evaluating your relationships, look both at the depth of the ones you have as well as the variety amongst them.

Basic Need #4: Personal Time

Even though relationships are important, we all need personal time as well. Literally never having a minute to yourself can cause your head to become overcrowded. You don't have any space to be alone with your thoughts. As a parent, it can feel like you have no time to be on your own. Your children need constant attention and so you never feel like you can truly take a break. But you need to find some time to do so every day, because these alone spaces are incredibly important for your mind. These are the times in which you process the things that have happened to you throughout the day and clear your head to be able to make important decisions. Thus, taking time for yourself isn't just something nice to do, it is actually a necessity in order to maintain your mental health. Some examples of personal time are journaling, going for a walk, meditating with the door closed. Whether you need to hire a babysitter or tag team with your partner, this alone time is well-worth the investment.

Basic Need #5: Professional Satisfaction

The final need we are going to talk about is professional satisfaction. Whether or not you have a job, you still likely have a sense of your own professional integrity. As a working parent, it can sometimes feel like a difficult push-pull between your workplace responsibilities and paying attention to your children. But this doesn't mean that you should completely let your professional life fall to the wayside. Caring about who you are professionally doesn't make you a workaholic, as long as you are able to leave that at the office. Applying for promotions, new jobs, or professional development programs can be incredibly personally fulfilling, giving you a stronger sense of your own abilities while potentially raising your salary. Who you are at work is who you are in the public sphere, the way that you give back to society, and so you should make sure to hold that dear and put energy into it. If you are a stay-at-home parent, you should also have aspects of the public sphere that bring you joy. Maybe you are involved with parent council at your child's school, volunteer with a local charity, run a side business, or even do something creative that you eventually want to do professionally, such as working on a novel. These things are just as worth investing in as a professional job, even if you aren't being paid. The main thing is that you have recognition outside of the family and feel a sense of competence and satisfaction with yourself. So, when you are considering your needs, don't forget that giving back to society, whether that's through your work or through other projects, is essential as well.

Self-Care: Treating Yourself

While the last section was all about making sure your basic needs were met, we are now going to pivot towards self-care, which takes these needs to a whole other level. Yes, you should make sure you are getting all the things you need out of life, but at the same time, most people want something more than just what they need. What is life without passions, adventures, and indulgences? It can be easy to get caught up in the needs and forget about the wants. When you are taking care of a child with a lot of needs, it can be hard to focus on your own needs, let alone the things that you want to do! But indulging in these things is actually incredibly important. In fact, self-care could be listed as the sixth basic need in the before list. Making sure your life is more than just a series of 'have-tos' is essential to making sure you have the motivation to keep going. Yes, you can achieve that through treating or rewarding yourself on occasion with an expensive purchase or vacation, but self-care is more than that. It's an opportunity to enrich your life and make it about more than the everyday. Here, we will talk about three types of self-care and give you some examples and strategies for integrating them into your life.

Things That Bring You Joy

The first kind of self-care we are going to talk about are things that bring you joy. This can mean anything from a favorite food to putting on an old album you loved in college to a night at the theater or a spa day. The most important part of this aspect of self-care is that it is something that brings *you* joy, not something you think should be enjoyable. If all it takes to completely relax you is a pint of ice cream, then there's no shame in that—go for it! If the thing that brings you joy costs a lot of money, then create a dedicated savings account for it and try to put away at least a dollar or two a day. That way, in a year or two, you can buy that plane ticket or expensive meal out without dipping into your main bank account! The key here is to find something that genuinely brings you joy in life and make it a priority, no matter your financial or lifestyle situation. Think of this as equally important as your physical health. Sometimes, even just looking forward to or planning the joyful thing can be a joy in and of itself! The happiness and personal satisfaction you get out of it will make you a better person, and in all likelihood, a better parent.

Things That Allow You to Express Yourself

Creative self-expression is one of the greatest joys in life. Since the beginning of time, humans have been expressing themselves through art, music, and stories. Nowadays, we have a more professionalized view of artistry, relegating creative expression to the people who do it for a living. But this doesn't have to be the way it is. Everyone is capable of expressing themselves, maybe not to a completely professional level, but certainly to a level that is satisfying to them and maybe those around them. If you have a creative outlet that you love, whether that be doing watercolor painting, singing, or anything else, make sure you make time to prioritize it. Maybe join or start a group of artists where you make deadlines for each other to make sure you are all making time for your creative expression. If you don't have a creative outlet, you should try exploring one. Think back to when you were a kid — what was your favorite creative subject in school? Finger painting? Music class? Playing make-believe? You can then bring these things into the adult world by pursuing life drawing, guitar lessons, or creative writing. Or look at your bucket list — what is something creative you have always wanted to try but never got the chance? Pottery? Tap dancing? Dressmaking? It's never too late to pursue these things and most major towns and cities have lots of affordable classes to try them out. Making time to either pursue existing creative outlets or experiment with new ones is a basic human need and something you should always prioritize in your life.

Things That Teach You Something

Many people romanticize their childhood or college years. Usually this is because you had less responsibility and the world was still very new to you, but another reason could be that you were learning a lot. You might have more responsibilities now and the world isn't so new to you, but the beauty of life is that you actually never have to stop learning! It's become a very trendy topic nowadays, the idea of the "lifelong learner," but it's actually very important to consider. There is so much to learn out there in the world and so why not take the time out of your life to learn some of it. There are so many different ways to learn so you can tailor it to your schedule as well. Maybe you have one evening free a week and so you can audit a night class at your local university. Or maybe you commute to work and can bring a book or a podcast with you on your commute, learning on the go! Or maybe you have a lot of housework to do, like folding the laundry. Instead of just flipping on the TV, put on one of the many free university lectures that are on YouTube. The most important thing to note here, like the other two sections, is that you pursue something you're genuinely interested in. No need to read famous authors that don't speak to your experience or learn about subjects that you aren't interested in. Find the subject or the genre that sparks your interest and challenge yourself to learn more about it. Like with your child's interests, which we talked about in the last chapter, you will be infinitely more motivated to continue pursuing them. Taking time out of your life to expand your mind is an essential part of life and can truly enrich your world.

Balancing Your Child's Needs With Your Own

Throughout this chapter, we have been reinforcing the idea that you deserve to prioritize your own needs. But of course, that isn't always possible. If your child's health or safety is at risk, you absolutely don't want to be off at an evening class or journaling in your bedroom. At the end of the day, your child's immediate needs are going to trump your needs, and especially your wants. It's just about balancing the times when you are able to care for yourself and for your child. Timing is really everything in this scenario. There's no reason that you shouldn't have a fulfilling life, it's just about finding the right places to fill it in. Of course, emergencies happen, but they are the exception. You have the ability to create a life that leaves room for your self-care and health, you just need to find ways to do it intelligently. Here, we will give you some smart strategies for fitting your needs in between your child's.

Strategy #1: Choose Your Battles

Sometimes, the need you are talking about with your child is actually a rule you are trying to enforce. Maybe your child hasn't done their homework that night yet, but you don't have time to sit down and help them with it because you have to cook a healthy dinner for yourself and the family. Now, you could always order a pizza and sit down with your child to do their homework, but that would be sacrificing your health for their homework. In this case, you have to decide what is really more important. Think about how many times your child has skipped homework that week versus how many times your family has cooked a healthy meal and choose the one that you've missed less. It's all about making those judgment calls. Or maybe you have a yoga class you've already paid for, but your child asks for you to watch a movie with them that night. It's all about choosing which you think is more important in the long term. Sometimes, you can let your health go for a night, but other times you can just say "next time" and stick to your schedule. Just know that it isn't the end of the world on either end and not everything needs to be a battle.

Strategy #2: Use Your Child's Away Time to Your Advantage

Unless you homeschool your child, it's likely that they are out of the house on most days. You might work for most of this time, but if you don't, either because you are a stay-at-home parent or because your job doesn't have nine to five hours, then you should absolutely use this time to your advantage. Say you don't work Tuesdays. Instead of spending that day doing general housework that you could do while your child is home, take advantage of the free childcare and schedule a pottery class for yourself, or audit a university course on that day. Blocking in things that you can *only* do when your children are being taken care of means that you will be able to do things that you wouldn't ordinarily feel that you have time to do. Those moments are incredibly useful for parents because they allow you to carve out time for yourself without disrupting your child's life or breaking the bank. It's a win-win!

Strategy #3: No Shame in Asking for Help

If you do work a nine to five, or you want to do something that only runs on the evenings and weekends, you should still find a way to do so. If you are co-parenting with a partner, arrange a tradeoff where you each get one night of the week to do something for yourself. Maybe your partner wants to do an evening fitness class and you want to try tap dancing. Agree that you will each have a "fun night in" with the kids on the others' respective night so that you can have equal access to personal time. Or, if you want to do something together, or are a single parent, there's no shame in hiring a babysitter or asking a family member to look after your child every week. Many babysitters like the regular schedule of a weekly gig and doing so will allow you to budget for it more frequently. You get a night to yourself, your kids get to spend time with another adult role model who can teach them different things, and so everyone is happy!

CHAPTER 5:

DEALING WITH OUTBURSTS

Probably the most difficult thing you will have to deal with as an ADHD parent are the outbursts. All children have outbursts, especially children in the toddler age group, but children with ADHD tend to have them more frequently and experience them more intensely. These can be extremely emotionally intense for your family. Your child is suffering, yet they are also taxing on your nerves as well, and so no one is feeling good. What's more is that there tends to be a strong stigma around children's outbursts, especially when they happen in public. No one wants to be the parent who has a screaming child at their feet at the grocery store, a family gathering, or, God forbid, an airplane. These outbursts are thus not only upsetting for the people involved, but can also carry a lot of shame around what people might think of you when they happen. That's a huge burden to carry and as the parent of an ADHD child, you don't need any more stress in your life. In this chapter, we will talk about all things outbursts, finally breaking the silence around them and helping you to both smash the stigma around ADHD outbursts as well as learn some meaningful strategies for dealing with them when they arrive. First, we are going to look at positive management methods for dealing with your child's ADHD outbursts, including more empathetic and child-led strategies for dealing with these outbursts. Then, we will pivot to the root causes of ADHD outbursts, which are almost always connected to unmet needs. And finally, we will talk about mitigating some of the stigma around ADHD outbursts, especially when they happen in public, but also when they happen on their own. Finishing the chapter, you should feel more confident going forward that you will be able to deal with your child's outbursts with more confidence and empathy and, most importantly, without shame.

Positive Management Methods

Most teaching and parenting involves some compromise between positive and negative reinforcement. It's a given that sometimes you have to give your kids punishments, even ones as minor as denying them dessert or a toy that they want, in order to teach restraint and consequences. However, when they are having an outburst, they are in a powerful state of emotional distress. More conservative wisdom would say something along the lines of "they need to suck it up," or "they're crying about nothing." But the more neurological research done about children's tantrums, especially those with ADHD, reinforce that it is actually positive attention that they need to come out of their outburst, not negative. Think about it this way, if you are having a terrible day and are generally irritable, what is going to take you out of that mood? Your partner or friend yelling at you and telling you to suck it up, or them telling you that sounds hard and offering to watch a movie with you? Yes, there are times for tough love, but in the throes of emotional breakdowns, it is a helping hand your child needs, not a reality check. Bringing your focus towards positive reinforcement strategies is such an important step for you to be able to actually bring your child out of their outburst and back into the real world. Plus, many positive reinforcement strategies can actually be teaching moments which not only help your child feel better in the moment but which actually help them to prevent outbursts in the future or be better at resolving them. In this section, we will talk about some of the best positive reinforcement strategies that will not only help your child to crawl out of their emotional outburst, but enact long-lasting change that will help build emotional tools they will retain for the rest of their life.

The Empathetic Approach

The first thing you need to do when your child is having an outburst is to have some empathy. It can be tempting to think only of yourself in the moment, which many people tend to do in an intense situation. Being in public or in the midst of work with a screaming child beside you is not a fun position to be in, and so most people are wont to focus on how upsetting the situation is for them. But what you really need to focus on is your child. They are the one who is causing this situation and so it is their mind you need to learn to understand. Throughout the past few generations, there has been a less empathetic attitude towards children. You might have grown up around such invalidating phrases as "children are meant to be seen and not heard," or "stop crying or I'll give you something to cry about." These kinds of phrases lack empathy for the child's emotional situation and reinforce the idea that the child is somehow deliberately trying to cause an outburst and is doing so for attention or out of spite. But what you have to remember is that children have the same frustrations, fears, and complexity of feeling as you do. Expecting your child to never have an outburst, especially when they are living with a condition as stressful as ADHD, is actually holding them to an impossible standard. You are essentially expecting something of them that you would never expect of yourself. For this reason, it's very important to try to exercise your empathy and remember that your child is not happy during their outburst either. Here are some ways you can think about this experience to help you to get into this mindset.

Strategy #1: Think of Your Worst Day

We've all had bad days, days where we had an emotional outburst, threw a tantrum, or acted out of turn in some way. While your child is having their outburst, try to think of the way you felt on your worst day. What was going through your head? What set you off? What did you feel like you wanted at that moment? Connecting with your past emotional frustrations can help you connect much better with how your child is feeling and help you deal with them more intuitively.

Strategy #2: Remember Their Lack of Agency

As we have mentioned several times throughout this book, children lack the kind of agency that you have. When you feel tired, you can call in sick to work, cancel dinner with a friend, or go to bed early. Children are not offered that same level of agency over their lives, with adults constantly scheduling them and often not letting them skip out on things. Your child has to push through being tired a lot in their life, which is something a lot of people can relate to. So when you see them having an outburst, this is often their only method to express their fatigue or discomfort and can even be seen as a strategy for reclaiming agency when they don't feel like they have it.

Strategy #3: Do A Necessities Check

We will talk about this later on in the chapter, when we discuss the relationship between outbursts and unmet needs, but there is an important place for the role of examining your child's needs when they are having an outburst. Think back to the rest of the day. Did your child get enough sleep last night? Did they have a filling and healthy breakfast? Have they been walking more than they usually do? Is it very hot or cold out? Are they drinking water? Have they not had very much downtime? Going through a simple checklist of things that might be contributing to the outburst can help you understand where it's coming from. Children, especially younger ones, often don't think about their day in this way and so likely won't understand why they are upset, but you can do some simple sleuthing to figure out what is going on. It might just be a matter of moving to a shadier spot, getting your child a small snack, or letting them sit for a few minutes to get them to calm down. They aren't always able to figure out their needs, but you can certainly try to do so for them!

Child-Led Resolution

The other way that you can create positive methods of outburst resolution is through putting your child in the driver's seat. Even though, as we talked about in the last section, they might not always be consciously aware of what they need, they will be intuitively aware. When your child is having an outburst, notice their body language and what they are tending towards. If they stop in the middle of the street while walking or sit down on the ground, it is likely because they are tired and their body is giving out. Or, if they seem to be constantly sheltering their head, it is likely too sunny for them and making them uncomfortable. With the empathetic approach, you would attempt to remedy these things right away, but with the child-led approach, you can simply use these observations to prompt questions. You can ask them what they want to have happen. You might find that, even though they aren't immediately consciously aware of what they are feeling, they are actually responsive when you prompt them. Try asking questions like "do you want a snack?" or "would you like to sit down for a few minutes?" to get them to consider what they need. Of course, they might be a little too far gone in their outburst to really think clearly, at which point you should revert to a different approach. Thus, the child-led method actually works best when they are in the early stages of a breakdown, when you start to notice discomfort. This approach can be used to stop outbursts before they happen.

Teaching to Self-Soothe

Throughout childhood, we have our parents to help soothe us, giving us positive reinforcement, comfort, and whatever else we need to overcome emotional issues. But as we get older, we are increasingly met with situations where we don't have our parents, or really any support system, in our vicinity. In these cases, we have to do something called 'self-soothing.' Self-soothing is a practice wherein people de-escalate themselves. Instead of having a parent say reassuring things or offer support, you are able to do so yourself. Now, obviously everyone needs support sometimes. No one can go their entire lives without experiencing support from others. However, you will need to learn how to do some amount of self-soothing for in-the-moment instances of distress. Maybe you are in line at the bank and start to feel anxious, or driving on your own to a job interview. If you are unable to access help from others, you need to know how to self-soothe in these scenarios.

In the case of children, they generally don't have good self-soothing skills. These things develop naturally as we age and are on our own more and more. But for children with ADHD, learning to self-soothe earlier than other people is very important. They are going to experience a lot more emotional distress than the average person and it will be very helpful for them and others to learn how to self-soothe as early as possible. In this section, we will give you some important self-soothing techniques that you can teach to your children to help them to learn how to self-soothe.

Technique #1: Five Senses Check-In

One self-soothing technique that is often used for people who are experiencing disorientation, distress, or dissociation is the five sense check-in. This is a calibration exercise that helps you to orient yourself in the world. It is related to the concept of mindfulness, which is all about connecting you to the outside world and noticing the small things. Thus, the five sense check-in works to both distract you from your issues by giving you a focus and to help bring you back down to reality when your mind might be racing. The technique works like this: You have to find five things you can see, four things you can touch, three things you can hear, two things you can smell, and one thing you can taste. This can be done either stationary or by physically going around a room. This exercise reconnects you with your senses and can be very calming and effective for people when they are having an outburst. Try running this exercise with your child when you notice them in distress and encourage them to do it themselves. Eventually, they will hopefully think to do this exercise unprompted, even when you are not around. If this exercise proves effective for them, they might continue to use it throughout their life when they are experiencing distress.

Technique #2: Breathing Regulation

When we become anxious, our vitals go up, meaning our heart rate and breathing in particular. This is an evolutionary response to help us escape from predators, but it can prove very difficult to stop it once it starts, causing anxiety that is more prolonged than it needs to be. When your child is having an outburst, it is likely that their heart rate is through the roof and they are hyperventilating. One important way they can calm down is to consciously regulate their breathing. Conscious slow breathing helps bring down vitals, sending a signal to the body that the threats have passed. There are many different breathing techniques to try, but one of the most common ones is five second breath in through the nose and ten second breath out through the mouth. This helps slow your breathing to a relaxed state and calm you down on a chemical level. Start to do some of these deep breath exercises with your child when they are having an outburst, or even after the fact, to help bring their body's anxiety down to a manageable level.

Technique #3: Relax the Body in Stages

It's one thing for people to say to you "just relax" but another thing altogether to be able to actually do so effectively. One of the reasons for this is that the body is simply very large. The brain is built to send signals to specific body parts and so when you ask it to relax every single part of the body, it has trouble doing so effectively.

This is why breaking down your body into parts to relax individually is so effective—it is hijacking the brain's intuitive signaling system. To do this exercise effectively, you need to break your body down into parts. One technique is to go from the toes to the crown, naming every body part you can go up your body. As you name them, your brain will naturally focus on that body part and have a much easier time relaxing specific muscles. This exercise can be done alone or aided by another person. You can start by directing your child through this exercise. Get them to lie down on the floor and speak in a soft voice, leaving 30 seconds to a minute of space for concentration in between each body part. "relax your toes… relax your feet… relax your ankles… etc." Like the other exercises, if this is an effective one for your child, they should ideally be able to eventually do it for themselves. Through these three techniques, you can teach your children meaningful strategies for self-soothing.

Outbursts as Unmet Needs

In an earlier section of this chapter, we talked about doing a check-in for the possible discomforts your child might be facing. Here, we are going to go into that in a bit more depth. When your child is experiencing distress, it is almost certainly because one of their needs is going unmet. If you think back to all the outbursts you have had in your life, even as an adult, it becomes clear that these must have been due to some kind of unmet need. Maybe you were overworked, or experiencing tension in your marriage, or not getting enough exercise. These kinds of things can be momentary, affecting just one day of your life, or they can be ongoing, creating years of piling up irritability. In all likelihood, if you have ever gotten therapy or simply talked to a friend, you know how liberating and validating it can be to identify the source of your distress. To be able to say out loud what is bothering you deep down can sometimes even make the problem go away, or at least drive you closer to a solution. For example, you might be irritated all day, never seeming to get along with anyone and not realize the reason. Then, you might remember that you forgot to eat breakfast and you are actually just hungry. Once you have a sandwich, you realize how much better you feel. This is a simple solution, but in many cases, emotional volatility actually does have a simple solution. If you extend this same logic to your child, you will realize that most of their outbursts are rooted in either some form of discomfort or unmet emotional need. If you are able to identify this need or discomfort and help your child identify it as well, then you will be able to find much more effective solutions for your child's outbursts. In this section, we will talk about how to identify and offer solutions to these unmet needs, as well as some of the common unmet needs ADHD children face.

Opening Lines of Communication

The first thing you need to do is open lines of communication. When it comes to communication between parents and children, it is all about two things: safe spaces and emotional education. To the first point, you need to create a space where your child feels comfortable sharing with you. This can be something as simple as needing to go to the bathroom or something as complex as feeling like they aren't being heard. If you react too often with hostility when your child expresses this to you, then they won't view you as a safe space where they can express their feelings and unmet needs. You should always react with openness whenever your child shares something with you so that they know that they can always go to you and don't have to fear shame or rejection. To the second point, you need to help your child build a strong emotional vocabulary. Many adults go their entire lives without being particularly emotionally literate, which means that they don't develop the important tools to recognize their needs and whether they are being met. If you want your child to be able to deal with their intense emotions in a mature way so that they don't turn into outbursts, then you need to teach them these emotional tools. Ask them questions like "what kinds of things are going through your head during an outburst?" or "what color would you use to describe your feelings?" to help them start to identify their inner thoughts better. Through these two strategies, you can help to build your child's communication skills, giving them a person to communicate with as well as the skills and vocabulary to do so effectively.

Common Unmet Needs

Every child is unique, but there are some certain unmet needs that are more common than others. You know your child best, and you know what they tend to feel, but you also should have in your back pocket a list of some of the things that they might be experiencing. This list can work as a guide for you to navigate your child's emotions as well as a sort of laundry list for you to run through if you are truly at a loss for what is bothering them. Here, we will talk about some of the most common categories of unmet needs that your child might be experiencing.

Physical Needs

Sometimes, the answer really is something very simple. If your child is having an outburst in public, they really might just be experiencing an unmet physical need that they are having trouble expressing. This might be hunger, thirst, overheating, exhaustion, needing to go to the bathroom, or anything of the like. It might seem like a simple thing and you might wonder why they didn't just say so, but we don't always realize when we are feeling these things. As we stated in an example from the last section, you might forget to eat and not realize why you're grumpy. Kids and adults alike experience this, so no need to fault your child for not using the bathroom at home or finishing their breakfast when they had the chance. We're all human and we all make mistakes like that. Your best course of action is to remedy the situation as soon as possible. One good strategy is to keep a kit on hand with some healthy snacks like granola bars or fruit, always have water, and always have a bathroom or rest plan. These tricks in your back pocket can often nip an outburst in the bud and help your child to meet a need they might not have even known they had.

Emotional Needs

Slightly more complex are emotional needs. Your child might seem like they are less experienced or complex than you are, but the level of emotions they feel is just as intense. Something that might not be a big deal to you might mean everything to them. Maybe not getting to go to a movie they wanted to see seems like nothing to you, but it was something they were looking forward to all week and emotionally, it would be the same thing as if your big vacation got canceled or you didn't get to go to your best friend's wedding. Kids feel things often more intensely and so you have to be mindful that smaller things can set them off and they might need emotional care for something that you wouldn't. Some of the most common sources of unmet emotional needs in children are lack of attention or feeling ignored, not feeling like their voice is being heard, feeling like they have no say in what happens, or feeling blamed for something they don't feel like they have control over. Recognizing that your child has these needs and that if they go unmet, they might result in an outburst, can help you to construct an environment in which they always feel like they are heard, recognized, and considered. Hopefully, assuring them of this during a breakdown can help in the short term and prioritizing these needs daily can help in the long term.

Stimulation Needs

Children with ADHD have unique needs when it comes to stimulation or lack thereof. Feeling over or under stimulated can thus actually be very distressing for your child. If they are in an environment with any kind of extremity, be that noise, light, temperature, crowds, etc. they are vulnerable to over stimulation. On the other hand, if they are in an environment in which they have nothing to occupy themselves, they run the real risk of being understimulated. If your child is having an outburst in a certain environment, you might want to think about the circumstances of that environment and whether it might be contributing to the outburst, especially if they have had an outburst in that kind of environment before. Are there flashing lights? Loud noises? Lots of people? Or on the other hand is there nothing to look at? Does your child have no one to talk to or nothing to read? Is there no window to look out of? Considering the circumstances of the environment can help you to really investigate where your child's outburst might be coming from and amending or removing them from that environment can be a highly effective solution for said outburst.

ADHD Accommodations

For children with ADHD, there need to be specific accommodations made in any environment or task. One of the worst things you can ask a child with ADHD to do is perform to the same level as a child without ADHD in the same environment and expect them to thrive. Their brains are inherently working differently from the other people in their vicinity and so they simply won't be able to. But if they are continually expected to perform at this level, they might start to build up lots of frustration and resentment. This can happen at school in relation to classmates, but it can also play out at home. If you have other children who don't have ADHD, you might experience some frustration that your ADHD child cannot do the same things in the same way, or sometimes needs extra help. They are aware of this and it likely makes them feel really ashamed and frustrated with themselves, which can lead to outbursts. Your job as a parent is to first manage your own expectations and then subsequently make sure your child knows that you don't expect the same things from them as you would from another child. Changing expectations and getting your child the accommodations they need can help you to create an environment in which your child feels accepted, validated, and in control.

Overcoming the Shame

Let's go back to the image of the screaming child in the grocery store. You're in the produce aisle, just trying to get the shop done as soon as possible before you have to pick your other child up from daycare, and your ADHD just isn't having it. They're at their wit's end and they completely break down in the store in front of everyone. You can feel all eyes on you as you try everything to calm your child down, but nothing seems to work. Eventually, you just leave the store and go back to the car, abandoning your cart of unpurchased produce—at least in the car no one has to hear your child scream. Once you're out of the situation, you start to beat yourself up. *Why didn't I handle that better?* You might be asking yourself, *I remember seeing parents with screaming kids before and thinking that they must have no idea what they're doing. Now I'm that person!* These negative thoughts can be really damaging and can make you feel like you have failed as a parent. But there's no need to feel this way. With ADHD, and even without, outbursts like this from children are to be expected and often have no easy solution. Here, we will give you some tips on how you can reduce shame and judgment around these outbursts.

Tip #1: Break the Ice

One of the most embarrassing things about a public outburst is the blank stares from others. But if you turn these interactions from silent judge and silent judge-ee into a plea for sympathy, you can reduce some of that judgment. You could make eye contact with someone and apologize, saying "I'm so sorry, my child has ADHD and has had a long day, we're going to take a break," or "I hope we aren't disturbing you, we're going to go cool down outside." Just make sure you don't hurt or trivialize your child's feelings in the process. This can help others understand where you're coming from and maybe have more sympathy for your situation.

Tip #2: Be an ADHD Advocate

This one can be done in either the short or the long term, but what you essentially want to do is help educate people on ADHD and how it works so that they are also more understanding when they see your child having an outburst. In the moment, you could say something like, "My child has ADHD and is really overstimulated right now, which is common for their condition, she needs to get to a quieter place." This identifies your child's condition, as well as the major symptom that is contributing the most to the current situation, and explains the solution you are about to take. Again, people are more likely to feel sympathy for you if you explain what is happening and what you are doing about it. In the long term, you can raise awareness around ADHD in your local community, perhaps starting a social media account spreading facts about the condition or starting a support group for local children. These efforts can help raise awareness for ADHD in general, meaning that the average person will be less likely to judge you if they witness an outburst from your child. Both of these strategies help you to make it clear why your child is experiencing outbursts and make those around you understand ADHD.

LEAVE A REVIEW

As an independent author with a small marketing budget, reviews are my livelihood on this platform. If you're enjoying this book so far, I'd really appreciate it if you left your honest feedback. I love hearing from my readers, and I personally read every single review.

CHAPTER 6:

TEACHING EMOTIONAL REGULATION

People with ADHD, especially children, tend to struggle a lot with regulating their emotions. They don't feel like they can express things to the degree that others can, nor do they feel like they can truly hold back when they are experiencing too-strong emotions. One of the reasons for this is that children with ADHD tend to struggle with "feeling through" their emotions. Feeling through emotions is a facet of emotional intelligence, something people are realizing more and more is necessary for a healthy emotional life.

The Importance of Feeling Emotions

In contemporary American culture, we are starting to see a shift in the way we think about emotions. In the past, there was a stronger culture of emotional repression, especially within parenting. Parents would prioritize getting their children to stop crying or training them not to cry in the first place over finding out why they're crying. This culture prioritized toughness and a stiff upper lip over empathy and investigating issues. There might be a few reasons for this. In times of hardship, people often have to forgo their emotional needs in favor of practical concerns. Your parents or grandparents probably grew up during the depression or world war two, times where they would have experienced material scarcity and insecurity. But we don't live in those times, and we can now focus more intently on the ways in which emotions manifest in complex ways. Unfortunately, many people still live, even subconsciously, under this kind of repression, being unwilling or unable to express their emotions to others. If you have a child with ADHD, it's imperative that you allow them to feel their emotions fully and help them to work through them in a way that develops emotional intelligence. Otherwise, they may end up repressing their feelings.

So why is repressing feelings bad? I mean, isn't it a good thing to not have to think about all of your problems every single second of the day? Isn't it somewhat of a relief to bury the things that bother you the most so you can focus on the positives? Well, yes and no. While you should not be ruminating over your problems all day every day, you should still be making space for your feelings. There are a lot of dangers that come along with repressing emotions too much, which you will start to see in your children if you don't work hard to teach them emotional regulation and intelligence. Here, we will look at some of the most important consequences of emotional repression, both for yourself and for your child.

Reason #1: Repression Prevents Progress

The biggest disservice that you do to yourself and your child when you repress is you prevent yourself from ever growing as a person. Think back to the times when you experienced the most growth and learning. Often it was when you confronted a difficult truth about yourself or finally admitted something out loud for the first time or acknowledged that someone hurt you. These big emotional breakthroughs can actually be really groundbreaking for your sense of self. They push through your existing narratives and get you to see who you are from a new perspective. They allow you to let go of lies you might have been telling yourself or things you might not have been able to acknowledge. When you take something difficult and push it down into the depths of your mind, you are essentially telling yourself that the pain or confusion you felt in that moment isn't worth acknowledging, which can be deeply invalidating. If you never deal with these things, you miss out on an opportunity to validate yourself, seek deeper truths, and come to terms with things that might be difficult or painful. When you do finally acknowledge these things, it might involve some initial pain. You might have to feel worse before you feel better, but trudging through this field of mud is necessary to get to the other side where you will certainly come out a stronger and wiser person. Having the strength to really feel your pain and look at it head on is a hard skill to develop, and a difficult thing to deal with, but it is definitely necessary in order to live an honest and fulfilling life.

Reason #2: Sharing Is Caring

One of the best things you can do for yourself is to develop strong and close relationships with other people. What this entails is to be vulnerable with them, to share sides of yourself that you might not show to everybody. What this also offers you is another person to comfort you when you feel pain, which can really help share the burden and make life's problems seem more bearable. Repressed people, however, cannot do this properly. Because the pain they have inside is not accessible to them consciously, it's impossible for them to be truly vulnerable with other people. As a result, they really struggle to build deeper connections and seek help when they need it. As a parent of a child who is going through a lot, you likely want them to be able to come to you with any problem they might have. This is very difficult to achieve if you have raised a child who is emotionally repressed. They will not know how to reach out to you, or even be able to recognize that they need to reach out. Going forward in life, they will also struggle to form close connections, always holding something back and never feeling like they have the space to share their pain. If you want your child to be able to share the deepest parts of themselves with others and receive emotional support from you and anyone else in their life going forward, then you need to make sure they are well-versed in emotional expression.

Reason #3: Feelings Always Come Back

The last major reason that repression is bad is that it simply doesn't work. No matter how hard you try to ignore your feelings, they are still in there deep down. And the funny thing about repressed feelings is that they will return no matter what. Even if you are not thinking about them consciously, they are going to have an effect on your life. Whether you like it or not, they will come out. Some common symptoms of repressed emotions are irritability, emotional instability or volatility, an inability to broach any subject related to the feeling, and even physical pains like migraines or muscle tension. Your body, or even your subconscious mind, always remembers everything that happens to you and will continue to remind you of it if you choose not to confront it. At the end of the day, repression is merely forcing your subconscious to deal with things that you really should be dealing with in your conscious mind. If you aren't able to move past these feelings, they will only continue to grow and take over your life on a subconscious level.

Types of Repression

Another thing to remember is that not all repression is made equal. Repression is going to look different for everybody. Some people will be evasive with deeper talk, but still see people. Others will avoid social contact altogether. But one big distinguishing factor in repression is how the repression starts. Most of the time, especially in adults, it will be self-enforced, but there is also a lot of repression-encouraging language that parents tend to use. It's tempting to do so. You don't like to see your children upset and so you try to nip it in the bud as soon as possible. Or rather, you are afraid of your child becoming soft and so you encourage them to toughen up a bit. Whatever your intention, however noble, it is possible you are actually encouraging your child to repress their feelings. And as we saw in the last section, there are a lot of possible ill effects that this can have. But have no fear: If you are able to distinguish the kinds of statements that are repression-encouraging, you can learn how to avoid them so that your child doesn't fall into the trap of repressing their emotions and being unable to articulate themselves emotionally. In this section, we will talk about some of the most common repression-inducing narratives that parents use on children, explain the kind of harm that they can cause, and offer some alternatives.

"Big Girls/Boys Don't Cry"

This is a very common one. In fact, you were probably told this as a child. It tends to be common in boys, which is why so many men struggle to cry past childhood, but it can also be done to girls as well. When you associate crying with weakness, or with being a 'baby' and repressing cries with being mature, that sends a very clear message to children: expressing emotions is bad and if I want to grow up, I need to learn to repress them. Weaponizing the idea of being a "big kid" is really powerful for children. They are so afraid of being thought of as a baby and so if you even remotely insinuate that they are being immature, that will induce a powerful emotional reaction. It also creates a narrative wherein they feel like they will have to express emotions less and less throughout their life as they mature and incentivize them to repress more to seem older. It also creates a narrative that emotional regulation means not feeling your emotions at all, which couldn't be further from the truth. Being able to feel through your emotions in an intelligent way is actually a sign of maturity and wisdom, while running from your emotions and repressing them is the easier choice. Banning crying or associating crying with immaturity or weakness creates a false connotation between emotional repression and wisdom. But most of all, banning crying just really makes children feel like their crying, and by extension, their emotions, are not something that should be seen by others. These things are unsightly and make others uncomfortable, even those that should be close to them in life. Telling your child not to cry will eventually make them stop crying around you or, even worse, stop crying all together, which is absolutely counter productive to emotional growth.

So what can you do instead when your child is crying? Well, one of the best things you can do is let them cry out for a bit. Crying actually has chemical value. When our brains overload with hormones because of extreme emotions, we have to physically leak them out through tears. Letting your child shed some of these excess emotions for a bit is very important. However, you shouldn't just let them "cry it out," let them know that you're there for them by holding them or sitting with them patiently. Tell them that it's okay to cry, and even say that you cry sometimes too. If you feel like they are working themselves up too much, you can talk them through some breathing exercises, which should ward off any excess crying or hyperventilation. This exercise lets your child know that you respect their crying and that you will always be there for them through their emotions.

Invalidating Language

When you go to someone for emotional support or advice, you are being extremely vulnerable. And the thing about vulnerability is that it will either go very well or very badly. Being well-received by someone when you put yourself out there is one of the best feelings in the world. It can allow you to reach new heights in yourself and your relationship to that person. But on the other hand, being poorly received when you put yourself out there is one one of the worst feelings in the world. If you show your innermost self to someone and they react with indifference or outright judgment, it can feel like some of the worst rejection possible – the rejection of your very self. So, when you do put yourself out there, you have to make sure it's with someone who is going to receive you well. For children, this is almost always their parents, or at least a close trusted adult. Their peers are not mature enough to counsel them emotionally and so you are quite literally all they have when it comes to this kind of support. When they come to you, you need to make sure you validate them and listen as much as possible.

So what does invalidating language look like and how can you avoid it? Well, any language wherein you are shutting the other person's emotions down or dismissing them could be considered invalidating. So, for example, saying something like "it can't be that bad, other people have it worse," would be an example of invalidating language. While it is important to keep perspective, it is also important to make sure that you are centering your child's feelings and not casting them aside. They can know that there is suffering in the world while still processing their own emotions. In fact, if you foster emotional intelligence in your child, it is likely that they will have higher empathy and thus be more attuned to the hardships of the world. Instead, you could say something like "people go through hard times, and it seems like this is one for you," or something more specific to their situation. Sometimes, simply repeating back what they are experiencing can be really validating. Another common invalidating thing is relating your child's problems too much to your own life. You might feel like the situation is similar to yours, but there is a very delicate balance, especially if your child has ADHD and you don't. They are likely having experiences that you simply do not understand and so you need to be careful about the way you handle it. Saying: "Oh yeah, that happened to me too," and launching into a long story can make your child feel like you don't really care about what you have to say. Instead, you could say, "Yeah, that happened to me too, it's really hard, isn't it." This way, you are making sure they know you relate, so they are not alone, but still centering them in the conversation and inviting them to keep talking. If you use these strategies for centering your child and making sure they know they are being heard, you can assuage some of that harmful invalidating language.

Toxic Positivity

The final type of repression-inducing attitudes is toxic positivity. This might sound like a bit of an oxymoron to you. How could positivity, which is good, be toxic? Well, positivity in general is good. You should always try to look on the bright side of the situations you are in. It can help you gain perspective and reframe narratives about things. But there reaches a point where positivity is actually just covering up a dark interior, becoming more like repression than optimism. More recently, many people in our culture are starting to discuss how positivity at all costs can actually have a negative effect on people. It can cause people to create a veneer of "everything's fine" while inside they are actually suffering. Putting this on your child can actually have negative consequences for them. If you greet their feelings with phrases like: "Well, it will all turn out alright," or "That's not so bad if you really think about it," you are essentially telling them that their feelings aren't that difficult, making them feel crazy for being so upset. The truth is that bad things happen in life, even to your children. You might not want to think about it, but your children are going to experience pain in their life, pain which will feel very powerful and real to them. Telling them that they aren't actually feeling pain is doing nothing but shutting down the way they feel and invalidating their feelings. When it comes to positivity, make sure you put a limit on it.

How to Promote Healthy Release

Now that we know all about how repression works, why you should avoid it, and all the forms it can take, it's time to take a look at how you can start to teach your child about healthy emotional habits. Depending on the age of your child and their personality, they will likely have different needs when it comes to releasing their emotions. Thinking back to Chapter 3, where we talked about your child's distinctive qualities in relation to ADHD, you need to also think about the distinct ways in which they can then channel their emotions in relation to their personality. These things are called emotional outlets and can be great ways to channel negative emotions in both the short or long term. You might even have an emotional outlet. Ever feel better by doing yoga after a stressful day? Or writing in your journal? Those are emotional outlets! Again, everyone is different in what they like, but it's still good to have a list of some of the most common emotional outlets. In this section, we will talk about some of the best ways that you can help your child channel their emotions, breaking the techniques up into verbal, physical, and creative channels.

Verbal Channels

The first type of emotional outlet channel that we will be dealing with here are verbal channels. Verbal channels are essentially "talking it out" or finding ways to use words. This is the most direct way to help your child as it involves clearly discussing the problem or frustration they are having. These techniques are great because they can help your child get things off their chest while also developing their emotional and verbal skills. Here are some good verbal techniques to help your child channel their emotions.

Technique #1: Daily Check-Ins

A more preventative measure, daily check-ins are a great way to build emotional communication into your routine. This is also a good practice because children don't always know when they have something to discuss. They might not have the emotional intelligence to say to themselves: "That experience at school today really made me feel bad about myself, I'd better go talk about it at home tonight." But if you prompt them, then they might actually open up and begin to hash out an emotional experience they didn't even realize was important. Some phrases you can use during this check in could be: "Did you feel happy to be there at school today?" or "Are you feeling more tired than usual?" These kinds of questions prompt clear responses and help you to gauge how your child is feeling. This is a particularly important technique to practice while your child is undergoing ADHD treatment, as their symptoms are likely going to be experiencing a massive overhaul. Make sure to pay careful attention and provide lots of check-ins during this time, since there can be a lot of frustration.

Technique #2: Talky Time Outs

Time outs are a common punishment, or at least de-escalator, for parents. On one level, they can work great, giving your child some time to reflect on their actions and gauge whether they might have done something wrong. On the other hand, though, they can cause rumination, or make your child fester in self-pity. Why not try the "talky time out," a time out where you pull your child aside and have a little emotional check-in. If they seem to be acting out or being particularly irritable, take them aside and give them space to share anything with you they might want to share. You might be surprised by how they open up when you give them this space. Think of this as more of an as-needed check-in, where you ask them similar questions on an as-needed basis.

Technique #3: Role Playing

If you know about a particular experience your child has had over the course of the day that they are upset about, then you can offer them support about that. If it is a conflict with another person, sometimes doing some role playing can help your child access feelings that they didn't even know they had. Try playing the role of their friend and get them to say to you what they want to say to them. Or, you could even reverse the roles, you playing the role of your child, and asking them to imagine what they think their friend might say to them. These little exercises can help your child articulate feelings they might not say to you directly and can even be a practical device for practicing apologies and the like. Try this if your child is having trouble with articulation or if they have a direct conflict.

Physical Channels

Although we might think of verbal outlets as the healthier option, associating physical outlets with aggression, there are actually some very positive and highly beneficial physical outlets for emotional frustration. Some people even attribute emotional frustration to lack of exercise. Remember back in Chapter 2, when we said that children needed at least 60 minutes of physical activity a day? Well the grim truth is that less than a quarter of American children actually meet this requirement. (*CDC | Physical Activity | Facts | Healthy Schools*, 2020) This obviously has massive physical and mental health consequences. You might find that, especially if your child is not meeting this threshold, physical activity is just what the doctor ordered.

Physical activity keeps your mind and body healthy, boosts your mood, and builds strength. It also uses energy, which means that negative emotions can be channeled into it, making it an ideal activity for kids that have a lot of pent up negative energy. Here are some important physical activities your child can do to make sure they are getting enough exercise.

Technique #1: Shaking It Off (Literally)

Sometimes the body just needs to let off some short-term steam. Do you ever feel that urgent sense of restlessness when you are particularly emotionally distressed? Well, sometimes just shaking your entire body, going limp and jumping up and down can help release a lot of that. Plus, it's something that kids love! They never get permission to jump around and go wild, so they'll definitely want to participate in this activity. Set a timer for thirty seconds to a minute and just jump and shake together. You'll be sure to feel refreshed and rejuvenated afterwards.

Technique #2: Dancing

Dancing is one of the best physical activities to do. For one, it uses your entire body and gets you to move in ways you might not ordinarily. Second of all, it's really fun, so you don't even realize you're exercising while you're doing it. And third of all, it stimulates your creative sensibilities and trains your musical and rhythmic brain. There's so much to be said for dancing, as it can be both a creative and physical outlet at the same time. If you notice that your kid is feeling anxious, try popping some of their favorite danceable music on the speaker and have a little dance party. You can even play a console game that involves dance steps to make it even more of a game. If you really get something out of it, you can even think about turning it into a fun family routine and continue to do it every week!

Technique #3: Yoga or Floor Exercises

Yoga might not be the first thing you think of when you think of kid-friendly exercises, but it's actually really easy for them to do. Kids are naturally flexible and so you might even find your kid out-stretching you, even if you're a regular yoga-doer! The good thing about yoga, pilates, and other low-impact floor exercises is that they have both a muscle-stimulating, but also calming properties. For this reason, it's actually suitable to do before bed, while high-impact cardio is not. Try introducing some easy yoga poses into your child's bedtime routine and start reaping in those calming properties. You might find that they fall asleep right away after those activities!

Creative Channels

As you have no doubt noticed throughout your life, creativity can be very soothing for the soul. There's nothing like expressing yourself through painting, writing, or even playing music when you are down. These expressions give us an outlet that is beyond words, putting our thoughts and feelings into visual or musical ideas. This can be a great way for your child to let out some of their emotions, especially if they are feeling over or understimulated, a common ADHD symptom. Encouraging your child to both take part in creative activities on a regular basis, or even redirecting them towards a creative activity when they seem distressed can be a great and even productive way for your child to channel their emotions. Here, we will give you some creative activities that can be a very soothing outlet for your child.

Technique #1: Writing

Kind of like the cousin to the verbal outlets, writing lets your child put things into words, but in a more private context. They are able to express themselves without fearing that someone will judge them and perhaps express ideas that they would rather remained private. It is imperative that if you encourage your child to have a journal that you make it extremely clear that it is for their eyes only, you will not be reading it. Make sure to hold yourself to that. Your child is entitled to their privacy and will get much more out of the exercise if they are confident no one is going to read it. Even if you have an older child or teen and suspect that they are doing something dangerous such as drugs or self harm, you should still never read their journal. It is best to just confront them directly to maintain trust and autonomy. If you wouldn't want your child to read your journal, don't read theirs. Having a completely private space to vent their frustrations is a very useful form of channeling emotions.

Of course, there's also creative writing, like short stories, poems, screenwriting, and things like that. You can also encourage your child to engage in this kind of writing. If they are "blank page shy" then you can always give them a prompt. Ask them to write you a story about an elephant who wants to become a pianist or about a girl who moves far away from home. These prompts can get the creative juices flowing and who knows, maybe down the road they will start to think of their own ideas and you won't even have to give them a prompt! Using writing, in whatever form your child chooses, to stimulate creative outlets is a great use of their time.

Technique #2: Visual Art

If your child is more visual, it might be a good idea to give them some visual art activities to do. This is a great category because it is so broad. It could mean setting up an elaborate finger painting station, complete with smocks and easels, in your home. Or, it could simply mean carrying around some crayons and a sketchpad to entertain your child on the go. You could even enroll your child in an arts and crafts after school program at your local library or community center, which can help them connect with other children as well as build their creative skills. Art is such a soothing practice that can really help your child visualize the world and themselves from their unique perspective. There are even some more specific visual art activities you can do in relation to particular difficulties your child is having. For example, if they are struggling with identity and self-esteem, you can get them to draw an interests-based self-portrait, which is a type of self-portrait that includes things your child likes and dislikes. This helps them to not only visualize how they look, but also construct a personal identity based on interests. From both a soothing psychological perspective and a personality-building perspective, visual art can be a very productive emotional channel for your child.

Technique #3: Music

Often called the "food of the soul" music is one of the most foundational of the arts. Many parents enroll their children in piano or guitar lessons because they want to help their children build a musical sensibility early on in life. And this is for a good reason: Music is not only an enriching part of life, but also a stimulating thing for the brain. Learning music from a young age can actually make you smarter. But more than that it can also be a very important emotional outlet. Playing an intense piece on the piano can really let out a lot of frustration and leave you feeling purged afterwards. But don't worry if you haven't signed up your children for piano lessons yet, or can't afford to do so, there are plenty of opportunities to enrich your child's life musically. Putting on some favorite songs on the speaker and singing along to them as a family can be very fulfilling. You can even encourage your child to write their own songs. You can also try to learn a very easy instrument like the ukulele, perhaps even doing so alongside your child for an extra bonding exercise. Through all these avenues, you can help your child channel their emotions in a positive way.

CHAPTER 7:

HEALTHY HABITS
IN THE HOME

The kinds of things you do every day that tend to recur throughout your life are known as habits. Habits are the things that we reinforce in ourselves and tend to keep doing because we've been doing them for a while. For this reason, habits can both be very useful, but also dangerous. Fostering good habits in our lives is one of the best things we can do to have happiness and health. Falling into bad habits, on the other hand, can completely destroy your life and send you into a run of unproductivity. For kids with ADHD, habits are especially important. Since ADHD tends to encourage the development of bad habits, it's imperative that you make sure your children are practicing positive behaviors at all times. As a family, you need to be creating routines that encourage good habits and healthy behaviors. In this chapter, we will talk about how you can go about doing just that, creating a culture of healthy habits within your family. First, we will talk about the importance of habits, illustrating the power they have over people and how they can completely change your life. Then, we will talk more specifically about how habits affect ADHD, especially in children, and how they can be channeled towards ADHD recovery. Then, the second half of the chapter will be completely devoted to exploring different types of habits and some key habit-building techniques within those categories. Through the chapter you should learn valuable information about the promotion of good habits and gain skills towards making habits that help you and your child.

The Importance of Habits

So what's so important about habits anyways? Why do they have such a big impact on our lives? Well, the short answer is that our brains are hard-wired to form habits. Back in our hunter-gatherer days, human life was all about survival. We were just trying to get our next hunt or next meal, meaning that we had to act as quickly as possible and conserve as much energy as possible. This is why people tend to be motivated to take shortcuts when walking somewhere—to save energy—but also why we tend to take mental shortcuts as well. It might not seem like it, but the human brain actually uses up a lot of calories, meaning that using extra thoughts takes up valuable energy. Thus, the human brain has evolved to use its energy as efficiently as possible. When we do something more than once, the brain starts to think of it as a shorthand and starts to skip some of the intermediary steps required to get there. This is also related to the "neurons that fire together wire together" psychology. The more you follow certain thought patterns, the more they are apt to reaffirm themselves in your brain. And thus, a habit is formed.

You've probably noticed this automatic thinking pattern in your life before. Chances are, you don't have to remind yourself to do things that you do every day, such as brush your teeth or put on the kettle in the morning — it's second nature. Sometimes, this can work against you, like not being able to remember if you locked the door after you left for work because you lock the door so frequently your brain just did so on autopilot. But whatever the consequence of the habit, you know that the things you do every day tend to become second nature, not needing reminders. You might have also seen this habit psychology play out in your healthy or unhealthy habits. Maybe during summers you've noticed that your kids start to get up later and later, and as a result go to bed later and later, resulting in an unhealthy sleep schedule. This is an example of a bad habit. Or, maybe you've noticed that once you've done a morning jog seven days in a row, it seems easier to do it that eighth time because you've trained your brain to think it's normal. These examples of habit forming demonstrate how easy it is to develop good and bad habits, but also how hard it can be to break them.

The Habit Loop

One of the foundational principles in habit psychology is called the habit loop. The habit loop is a series of steps that construct habits in your brain. There are three main components to the habit loop: the cue, the routine, and the reward. These three steps comprise the main aspects of the habit. The first component, the cue, is the thing that triggers the habit. This could be a craving for a certain food, the desire to get fresh air, or the temptation to stay up late and binge on a TV show. The cue forms the motivation for the habit, and is reinforced through the next few steps. The next step is the routine, or the actual behavior. This could be eating the food, going out for a walk, or putting on Netflix. This is the actual thing that you are doing that forms the habit. And finally, there is the reward. For most bad habits, the reward is a dopamine rush or a release of stress, but for many good habits the reward is personal satisfaction or a sense of accomplishment. The reward might also be material, like earning money or weight loss. Whatever the type of habit, these three steps will play out in a loop, with the reward creating more motivation for the cue and continuing the cycle all over again. The key to breaking bad habits and encouraging good ones is to hijack this cycle and create a new loop that is more positive for your life. Being aware of the habit loop and how powerful it can be is the first step to reinventing your habits.

Hijacking the Habit Loop

So how exactly is this done? It seems from the previous section that this habit loop is difficult to break—how exactly do you do so? Well, it's not easy, but it can be done. The first step is to really examine the cue. What is the desire that is driving you towards the habit in the first place? To help your child break a bad habit, you should be asking the same questions. Is it the dopamine rush of eating a bunch of sugar? Is it the sense of relaxation that comes from spending all Saturday on the couch? Is it the relief from social anxiety when you cancel on a friend for the third time? These core 'id-based' desires are forming the building blocks of your habit and are essential to why the habit is happening in the first place. Once you consider and really evaluate the reason why you are partaking in this habit, you can start to unravel it. Here are some good strategies for eliminating unhealthy habits in your life.

The Redirection Method

One good strategy is to satisfy the cue by replacing the routine with something else. So, if you (or your child) tends to bail on social obligations because of fatigue or social anxiety, consider de-escalating the social situation. Instead of a party, have a movie night in with the friend. This way, you still satisfy the cue, but break the negative pattern with something positive. If your motivation is a sugar rush, try replacing the pack of chocolate chip cookies with a healthier alternative. You could make a naturally-sweetened smoothie or a chickpea-based chocolate chip cookie to still get that something sweet without all the empty calories. Doing these alternatives allows you to continue the cue, but also avoid the negative consequences of the routine.

The Root Cause Method

Another effective, albeit more difficult, strategy is to try to redirect the cue altogether. If you dig deeper into *why* you are feeling the cue, then it might help you address the root causes, rather than just the routine. Perhaps you or your child crave a lot of sugar at the end of the day because you feel low in energy and so you are craving a sugar rush to get your energy back on track. Perhaps all you need to do is lower other stress levels in your life or eat a more filling or healthier breakfast or lunch. Making these adjustments might actually eliminate the cue altogether. The root cause might also be emotional. Maybe you or your child are facing social anxiety because you feel like you're not interesting enough for other people, thus avoiding interactions out of fear of rejection. Getting help for this issue might start to eliminate that negative cue and thus help break the habit. Whatever the cause, finding a way to address the negative cue in your life can do a lot for your habits.

Responsibility as the Parent

Throughout this section, we have been implicating you as the parent quite a bit. You might be wondering why this is the case, since this is supposed to be a book about childhood ADHD, but there is actually a very good reason for this. In a family unit, children don't really have much autonomy. They don't decide what food is in the fridge, when bedtime is, or what kinds of social functions happen in the house. For the most part, children just go with the flow. What this means, however, is that your habits have a major impact on your children's habits. The time you do things at, the kind of food you keep around the house, and the kind of social life you organize for your children all have a direct impact on their life. You can even indirectly affect your children's habits through modeling your own habits. As we discussed back in Chapter 3, children look to you as their role model, and thus will mimic the kinds of things you do. If you have a tendency to binge on junk food when you're stressed, chances are your children will do the same. This is not to make you feel anxious, but to make you realize that the things you might be concerned about in your children are

146

also probably reflected in yourself. If you notice your child engaging in a negative habit, chances are you have also done the same thing. Sometimes, making the effort to change your own habit can have an impact on your child and help them to kick the habit too! Remember: You're all in this together as a family, so make sure that you realize the impact you all have on one another.

Habits and ADHD

One thing you are probably wondering about is the impact of this habit loop on the condition of ADHD. How do habits form differently around the condition of ADHD? Do people with ADHD make or break habits easier or harder than other people? Unfortunately, the Journal of Attention Disorders has found that children with ADHD are significantly more likely than other children to have bad habits. (*Are Kids with ADHD More Likely to Have Unhealthy Habits?* n.d.) Some of the negative habits that children with ADHD are the most susceptible to are unregulated sleep cycles, dehydration (inconsistent water consumption), and excessive screen time. These are typical grievances for parents in general, but they can be particularly pronounced in children with ADHD. The most difficult aspect of these findings is that not only do ADHD symptoms encourage these poor behaviors, but that these behaviors in turn make ADHD symptoms worse. Most ADHD research has found that having a regular sleep schedule, eating healthy food, drinking plenty of water, and limiting screen time (especially addictive screen time) is imperative for improving ADHD, as we talked about in Chapter 2. Thus, the tendency towards negative habits for children with ADHD is a negative loop that creates poor behaviors, then makes ADHD symptoms worse, which then makes the behaviors worse. For this reason, it is even more necessary than ever for children with ADHD to get the help they need and to start to break some of these patterns that are only making their condition worse.

Types of Habits

If you have a child with ADHD, it is likely they already have a whole host of unhealthy habits that they are relying on. And it's no wonder. Remember when we talked about the cue in the habit loop? Well, these cues are often based around some kind of unmet need or feeling of desperation. A child with ADHD growing up in a world without accommodations for their condition is certainly a person who is experiencing a lot of stress. They probably have a lot of fatigue and frustration driving them towards dopamine-inducing behaviors. But there's a chance that you aren't actually aware of the specifics of your child's bad habits. You might not realize the harmful things they are doing or even that you are doing as well. The first step to helping your child develop good habits is understanding the areas of life in which habits can form.

In this section, we will talk about different kinds of habits, what they look like when they are bad, and what you can do to try and improve them.

Nutrition Habits

The first kind of habits are nutrition habits. These are the kinds of habits you have around eating. We covered nutrition in Chapter 1, so you should have a good idea of your child's culinary needs. But it's one thing to know what your child needs to be eating and another thing to know when and how they should be eating it. You might have a healthy meal plan for your child, but what kind of snacks are available in your home? Does your child eat at consistent times throughout the day? Does your family make the effort to cook every night or do you tend to leave it to the last minute and order takeout frequently? These kinds of facts play a major role in your child's eating habits, not just the mealtime foods they eat. If you notice your child, or yourself, tending towards junk food binges, late night snacking, or putting off eating until late in the morning on weekends. So you should try to address what might be the cues that are instigating that behavior. From there, you can try to introduce more filling foods like healthy fats (think nuts and avocado) and plant-based proteins (think lentils and broccoli) into their meals so they don't crash so easily throughout the day, and maybe try some de-stressing exercises so your child doesn't feel the need to have dopamine hits through carbs and sugar. Implementing these changes will help your child to develop healthier habits with food and perhaps prevent crash eating.

Exercise Habits

So, you know that your child needs 60 minutes of exercise a day, but when exactly is that happening? Many people know that they are supposed to exercise, but simply feel like they don't have the time or have trouble fitting it into their schedule. If your child is busy, especially with after school activities that are sedentary, such as piano or art, then it can be really hard to find time for them to get exercise. Mornings are such a rush to get everyone out the door and they're so often tired after school, and by the time evening rolls around, you're already getting ready for bed and don't want to do any high-impact activities. So when do you fit it in? Well, one good strategy is to build it into your day. If you live walking or biking distance from your child's school (that is, under a 30 minute walk or 15 minute bike ride away), then you should try walking or biking at least once a week, if not every day. This not only builds walking into your routine, thus building a habit, but also takes time you would have spent commuting anyway and turns it into exercise time. If you don't live close enough to school, consider walking or cycling to one of your child's activities, such as piano lessons. Finding a place your child can walk or cycle to, perhaps even on their own if they are old enough, is a great way to build exercise into your routine and avoid the habit of the sedentary lifestyle that so many American families fall into.

Sleep Habits

One thing we haven't talked about too much yet over the course of this book is sleep. Nutrition and exercise are very important, but sleep is important too. And it's not just how much sleep you get per day, it's also the quality of sleep and the regularity of your sleep schedule. When it comes to the topic of habits, sleep schedule is a very important component to habit-building. Going to bed at wildly different times every day is actually one of the most harmful things you can do to your sleep schedule. Your body has something called a circadian rhythm, which helps you to naturally produce melatonin when you need to sleep and wake up in the morning feeling rested. If you are constantly going to bed at different times, then your circadian rhythm can't properly regulate itself. Staying up late, either to watch TV or to finish homework that was procrastinated, can be tempting. It can feel like sneaking extra hours off the day. But you need to learn to break this habit and put value into a consistent bedtime. Of course, there's no need to start mandating your children be in bed by eight o'clock — you should pick a time that suits your family's schedules well. The best way to calculate it is to work backwards from the time your children have to get up in the morning on a school day, subtract the amount of hours of sleep they need (from 8–14, depending on age) and then add an extra half hour for buffer. So, if your 12-year-old has to be up by 7:30 to catch the bus in time, and they need 9 hours of sleep, they should have a bedtime of around 10:00. You can push it maybe by half an hour on weekends, and perhaps an hour during the summer holidays, but maintaining a consistent bedtime, even when your kids don't have to be up that morning, will help them to regulate their circadian rhythms and build good habits around sleep.

Emotional Habits

Through the last few chapters, we have talked a lot about emotional regulation and building communication. These things are very important for your child with ADHD to build a path towards recovery. You might not think that this has to do with habits, but it actually does. Practicing emotional intelligence and communication on a regular basis is one of the best things you can do for your child. One good example of a good emotional habit is the daily check-in we talked about in Chapter 6.

General Lifestyle Habits

Other than the big four we talked about before, there are also lots of other things in your child's life that they can form habits around. These things can also be crucial to your child's physical and mental health and so should not be ignored either. Making sure your child has good habits in every single facet of their life is one of the most important things you can do. Here, we will look at three miscellaneous aspects of your child's life around which habits can also form. Through these three types of habits, we will also talk about ways in which you can improve and develop good habits from bad ones.

Homework Habits

First of all, it is an annoying reality that your child is going to have homework. Whether or not you agree with the concept of homework ideologically, your child is going to be expected to do it by their teacher and so they must find some way to do so. The difficult part is that your child is so often tired from doing schoolwork all day when they get home and the evening can very soon get away from you. For this reason, you really need to make sure that your child is making regular time to do their homework. Time management is a really important skill to develop and a lot of it comes down to habits. One good way to induce good homework habits in your child is to set a time that works for you every day and set an alarm on your phone for it. For children with ADHD, homework time might be filled with dread, causing them to delay it as much as possible. You can try to make homework a little easier or more fun by creating a designated "homework corner" with a little desk (kept consistently clear), snacks and water, and even calming music or white noise to improve concentration. Making sure that your child develops healthy habits around homework, especially relating to time management, is an important way to make sure they get those things done and continue those healthy habits throughout their life.

Socialization Habits

Everyone wants their children to have good friends, to create lasting bonds throughout their lives that will help them to grow as people. But for children with ADHD, socialization can be difficult. As we have talked about in previous chapters, children with ADHD are prone to social withdrawal, or even behavior that might cause them to be rejected socially. As a consequence, it might be difficult for your child to keep and maintain friendships, perhaps descending into loneliness, coming home every night and shutting themselves in their room. You might feel at a loss for how to get them out of their shell. One of the best ways to help your child socially is to construct a ritual around their social world. Instead of encouraging them to hang out with friends more, which may or may not happen, you should schedule regular intervals where your child has the opportunity to socialize, such as joining a club or doing an after school activity. Be sure to enroll your child in something that is both social and that they're interested in, whether that be baseball, knitting, theater, or dungeons and dragons. Whatever your child likes, enrolling them in something adjacent to their interests will both incentivize them to attend and also connect them more specifically to other kids they might have things in common with. Attending a weekly club is a great way to build a socialization habit that can benefit your child greatly, regularizing their connection and helping them connect with people they might relate to.

Screen Time

Ah, the dreaded screen. Every parent's saving grace and nightmare at the same time. On one hand, handing your kid an iPad or putting them in front of their favorite TV show can buy you valuable time to cook, clean, work, or enjoy something you like to do. But on the other hand, too much screen time for children is linked to mental health issues and at the very least, sedentary lives. While children used to be sent outside for parents to have alone time, the increasing fears around child safety as well as less walkable neighborhoods have brought American children indoors, the "sending outside" now becoming virtual.

While it is absolutely fine to allow your children some screen time (after all — think about how much *you* stare at a screen all day!), it is also important for this to be mitigated. TV shows for children and social media apps are designed to be addictive, dominating your attention with brain-hijacking algorithms that are intended to keep you hooked forever. While this makes a lot of money, it also is a nightmare for the child's brain, especially the ADHD child. Children with ADHD have a particularly difficult time regulating their attention spans, meaning that they are especially vulnerable to these algorithms that try to grab their attention. Thus, it is easy for them to lose track of time, perhaps spending an entire evening scrolling through Tiktok and forgetting to eat, do homework, or spend time with family. This is not to cause you to panic, but merely for you to recognize the value of limiting screen time.

One very effective tool to mitigate screen time is to set time limits. If your child is a TV addict, limit them to one or two episodes a night, depending on your family's schedule. If they struggle with gaming, social media, or any other app-based screen time, there are actually tools you can download. Some apps let you restrict the time spent on other apps, automatically shutting them down if you spend more than an appointed amount of time on them. So, for instance, if your child loves Tiktok, you could allow them 30 or 45 minutes a day on the app, which will then lock itself until the next day. This means that they still get to enjoy the content they love, while still being able to have time for other things. Making sure your child still gets to enjoy some moderate screen time, while also learning the value of knowing when to stop, is essential to responsible ADHD parenting.

CHAPTER 8:

EXECUTIVE FUNCTION: BUILDING COGNITIVE AND LIFE SKILLS

Back in Chapter 2, we talked about the brain and its functions. One of the biggest things we talked about was the prefrontal cortex. This is the part of the brain that is responsible for higher cognition and doesn't fully develop until the age of 25. Another word for this higher cognition is "executive function." Executive function is kind of like the central control board of the brain. It is primarily your conscious mind that engages in executive function, delegating tasks to the rest of your brain and creating the overall objectives the brain is working towards. Executive function is extremely important for ADHD. Even though your child does not necessarily have a functioning prefrontal cortex, they still have executive function. They will need to cultivate this executive function in order to successfully go through life productively. In this chapter, we are going to talk about some of the most important aspects of executive function. First, we will define executive function and break it down into its most essential qualities. Next, we will talk about the cognitive skills within executive function and the kinds of life skills that go along with them. Through this section, we will define four key cognitive and life skills that your child should work towards developing or improving on: Time management, focus, memory, and self-esteem. This chapter will help you to envision the kinds of skills children with ADHD need help developing from a more neurological perspective.

What Is Executive Function?

So, first of all, what exactly is executive function? How do we define the part of the brain that is responsible for these important tasks? You can think of your (and your child's) executive function as being responsible for those long-term planning goals. It helps you to override some of your base or dopamine-seeking behaviors and get on track with life's essentials. Basically, your executive function is the voice in your head telling you to do the dishes or get back to work instead of watching another episode of TV or scrolling through your phone. It is also the force that allows you to think ahead for your life, helping you to think about career goals, new hobbies you want to pursue, and all other kinds of higher goals. If you didn't have executive function, you would be meandering through life, with only short-term planning. One of the key features of executive function is that it contains three components: working memory, cognitive flexibility, and inhibitory control. Here, we will look at these three things together and discuss the ways in which they individually contribute to the overall purpose of executive function.

Working Memory

We tend to think of memories as being movie-like accounts of our daily life—our fifth birthday party, our prom night, our life-changing first trip abroad. These foundational memories as anecdotes from our lives are incredibly important, but working memory actually serves a slightly different purpose. Working memory is for things like to-do lists, reading, mental math, and things like that. It is related to short-term memory, but is even more practical, consisting of the easily-accessible information we need to use. Essentially, short term memory allows you to store information, while working memory allows you to use and manipulate this information. This is one of the most important aspects of executive function and begins developing as soon as we are born. In fact, you could reduce most of your daily brain activity to working memory. But working memory is not made equal in everyone. You have to really work to improve your working memory. Activities like mental exercises can vastly improve your working memory, creating a brain that is more apt to make judgements and calculations.

The working memory actually has two components: verbal working memory and nonverbal working memory. Verbal working memory consists of the conscious, word-based things that we remember. It is essential for developing reading comprehension skills and learning things in a typical school context. This is something that, if your child struggles with it, could be very dangerous. However, it is also the easiest component of working memory to exercise, so you should be certain that your child will be able to make improvements if they are struggling. Nonverbal working memory is everything else, such as visualizing images (or "the mind's eye"), doing math calculations, and spatial awareness. All of these things are related. They are not as based on memorization or conscious thought as verbal working memory. Both of these types of working memory collaborate to form the ways in which you practically think about the world.

Cognitive Flexibility

The second major part of executive function, cognitive flexibility, consists of the ability to adapt your thinking to different environments or contexts. So, let's say for example you are doing a math problem to learn about multiplication. You learn that if someone has three shopping carts of five apples each, they have fifteen apples altogether. When your teacher then asks you if there are five pig pens, each with three pigs, your cognitive flexibility kicks in. It allows you to recognize the intrinsic similarity between the two situations, even though they are in different settings and consist of different objects. Because your brain is able to transpose basic information onto different scenarios, you are able to solve the second problem easily. That is the fundamental function of cognitive flexibility.

Like with working memory, there are actually two basic components to cognitive flexibility: mental multitasking and modification. The first, multitasking, helps you to think of more than one thing at a time. This is not even necessarily as complex as "patting your head and rubbing your tummy at the same time," but even includes more basic things like talking while walking or chewing while reading. The second part of cognitive function, modification, is more akin to the way that cognitive flexibility was described before. Another example of this kind of modification-based cognitive flexibility is grouping. If you have a collection of students, there are many ways in which you could group these students. You could group them by age, height, hair color, favorite color, favorite animal, birth month, etc. If you are able to create different sets of groups amongst a collection, then you are putting your modification-based cognitive flexibility to good use. These functions help your child to learn new things, acquire new skills, and think about the world in new ways.

Inhibitory Control

One of the last aspects of executive function to form, and the one that people tend to have the hardest time with, is inhibitory control. Inhibitory control is what it sounds like—the ability to control or regulate your impulses. Impulse in and of themselves are not bad. Many of your impulses are actually necessary for your survival. The impulses to eat, go to the bathroom, and drink water are all necessary. Even more abstract impulses, like to go for a run, to take a trip, or to do something creative are all great and natural. However, we should also have the ability to evaluate our impulses and judge whether they are the right thing to do, or whether this is the right time to do them. For example, the urge to go to the bathroom is necessary, but if you are on a plane and the seatbelt sign is on, you will need to control that impulse and wait. Or, the impulse to take a vacation might be a good one, but if you can't afford it, you will need to control the impulse to buy a plane ticket that might send you into credit card debt. Thus, the idea of having impulses isn't inherently bad, but a healthy amount of impulse control is necessary to make sure that you stay on track in life.

Impulse control is a particularly difficult area for children and those with ADHD. You might notice that your ADHD child struggles to hold back certain impulses. Back in Chapter 1, we talked about things like interrupting others as a major ADHD symptom. This can be seen as a simple failure of the inhibitory control aspect of executive function. Instead of being able to control the impulse to say what they want to say and wait their turn, the child simply blurts out what they want to say. This is a clear ADHD symptom and sign that inhibitory control is lacking. You can start to help your child to improve their inhibitory control by discussing their impulses with them and coming up with a plan for what they should do if they have something to say and feel like they want to interrupt. For example, you could give them a pen and paper at the dinner table (if that's a place where they frequently interrupt) and tell them to write what they want to say down when they think of it, and then they can guarantee that they won't have forgotten what they wanted to say. Using strategies like this can help to improve your child's inhibitory control and their executive function in general.

Cognitive Skills as Life Skills

Now that you understand the basics of executive function, we can start to look at some of the more practical applications it might have on your life. When you are in the realm of neuroscience, it can all sound very impractical.

But the brain as an organ has clear implications on daily life, meaning that it will have noticeable effects on your child's daily life. Applying these things to the tasks your child has to go through in their life will help you to understand the steps they need to take for improvement. In this section, we are going to look at four foundational cognitive skills within executive function: time management, focus, memory, and self-esteem. These four important skills are not only necessary aspects of executive function, but also important skills that every child with ADHD tends to struggle with and should work on improving throughout their ADHD treatment.

Time Management

The first of these foundational skills is time management. We already talked a little bit about time management in the last chapter when we talked about habits, particularly around homework and screen time. Time management is a skill typically associated with maturity. Children don't really have a strong sense of time (ever asked your child to come down in five minutes? Not likely to happen) which is why they are so often heavily scheduled by the adults in their lives. However, with careful help, over time they should start to get an intuitive sense of time. But this is only the first step. Almost everyone, even if they have gained that intuitive sense of time, struggles to manage it. You'd be hard pressed to find an adult (especially a parent) who has not uttered the words: "there just don't seem to be enough hours in the day." Finding time to do things like housework, socializing with friends, hobbies, cooking from scratch, and getting adequate sleep can feel like an uphill battle even for the most time-conscious among us. Time management is thus a skill that almost everyone struggles with, but those with ADHD struggle the most. Because ADHD is a deficiency of attentiveness, children and adults alike who suffer from the condition lack both intuitive senses of time and the ability to schedule themselves and stick to it. For this reason, time management will likely be a lifelong struggle for your child, something you will have to help them with more than you would ordinarily.

Typical Struggles

The most common things that ADHD children struggle with when it comes to time management are hyperfocusing and sticking to schedules. Hyperfocusing is a common phenomenon within ADHD wherein the sufferer loses track of all other things but the task at hand, sometimes for hours on end, as we have discussed earlier in this book. Getting lost in hyperfocus is very common for those with ADHD, so it's important to help your child through that. Staying on track, and on schedule, is also something kids with ADHD struggle to do. They might get distracted and forget to do their chores, throwing off the whole evening, or take too long to finish their homework because of daydreaming and don't have enough time to watch a movie with the family. These schedule disturbances can be really frustrating for kids with ADHD, especially when it cuts into their other time. Helping them to stay on track is another key aspect of helping them improve their time management.

How to Help

There are two central components to helping your child through ADHD: check-ins and timer systems. The first, check-ins, are designed to help your child avoid hyperfocusing. Now, hyperfocusing isn't always bad. For example, on a Sunday afternoon when there's nothing to do, go ahead and let your kid read the encyclopedia for three hours or get lost in a coloring book. There's no harm in it. But if it is a school evening where you need to make sure homework, dinner, piano practice, chores, and bedtime rituals all get done, there isn't the same level of leisure time. If your child is hyper focusing too much on, for example, an aspect of their homework at the expense of finishing it on time, you need to make sure to check in. Sometimes a simple interruption can derail the hyperfocus. The second component is to set timers and not worry about tasks going unfinished. It's better for your child to have done half their homework, but still be able to eat dinner with the family and take a bath, than to finish it to the exclusion of all else. Get more comfortable with leaving things unfinished—when the timer goes, everything gets dropped! These simple strategies can help your child to stick to their schedule and start intuitively developing time management skills of their own.

Focus

Of course, the central issue of all ADHD is focus. However, due to the prevalence of hyperfocusing within ADHD, it is not necessarily teaching your child to be able to focus—they have no problem with that. It's simply the act of teaching them to control their focus. Similar to impulse control, children with ADHD really struggle to control when they are focusing on something intently and when they feel like they can't focus at all. This can affect their ability to do schoolwork, pursue hobbies, and even go through social interactions. Gaining control over focus is integral to mitigating ADHD symptoms and achieving a more productive mode of living. In this section, we will look at how the focus aspect of executive function helps your child live a better life.

Typical Struggles

The two major struggles for children with ADHD and focus is obviously finding a middle ground between hyperfocusing and lack of focus. Those without ADHD are able to maintain a steadier focus level, paying attention to what they need to pay attention to at the right time. Another aspect is the ability to force yourself to focus, even when you don't have too much vested interest or excitement about the thing you're looking at. This skill might seem like a really daunting task for someone with ADHD, but with the right kind of training, they can start to exercise their brains to have a healthier relationship to focus and perhaps try for a steadier relationship to focus in general.

How to Help

Training your brain to focus better is no easy task. One of the best things you can do for your ADHD attention span is to progressively train your attention. Find out how long your child is able to focus on their homework before they get distracted. Let's say it's five minutes. If this is the case, then you challenge your child to focus on their homework for six minutes. Because it's difficult to be able to tell the difference, they will likely find this pretty easy. Then, once they are comfortable with that, raise it to seven minutes. See how they respond to this and try to raise their focus time by a minute incrementally. Sooner or later, you might find that they're able to focus for more like ten or even fifteen minutes!

Another strategy is to eliminate as many distractions as possible and create a clear, dedicated workspace. Curate the space to be clear, to not have anything like books around that could be distracting. If your child is doing paper homework, remove all electronic devices from the room (laptop, phone, tablet, etc.). If they are doing work on the computer that doesn't require internet, turn the internet off on their computer while they're working, and if they require internet, try to set up temporary website blockers for the duration of their homework time so they don't end up on social media or gaming. You can sometimes even make these things password-protected so your child isn't tempted to break the rules. This might sound really harsh, but this isn't a full-time thing. You might only have to create these restrictions for 30 minutes per day, or however long it takes for your child to do their homework. Helping them to mitigate distractions around the house is a great way to get their brain used to focusing on just that task. Using these techniques can have a powerful long-term effect on your child, helping them to overcome some of their difficulty with focus.

Memory

Interestingly, many people with ADHD actually struggle with memory. It isn't necessarily that they struggle to hold onto memories, but more that they struggle to create memories while they are happening. See, memories actually require you to be paying attention to your environment in order to make them. If you are not present in the moment, then you will not be able to form proper memories. This is why you usually remember the bigger moments in your life, rather than specific days that followed your main routine—because you were more mentally present. Therefore, the way you need to help your child recover from memory issues is to help them be more present in the moment. Improving on the before categories, such as focus, will help them to make clearer memories and thus not miss out on a lot of the issues that come along with short-term memory loss and ADHD.

Self-Esteem

Having ADHD can be really frustrating. You are both running into problems with others as well as constantly feeling disappointed in yourself. Doing poorly in school, struggling to maintain friendships and hobbies, those things can all cause your evaluation of yourself to crumble. If you can't find a way to succeed in the way that society wants you to succeed, that is going to be frustrating no matter what, even if you have people building you up. This is especially true for those with undiagnosed ADHD, who don't necessarily have anything on which to blame their issues. Thus, many people with ADHD struggle with their self-esteem. It might not seem like self-esteem is a brain issue, but it actually is. Executive function, among long-term planning and important decisions, also affects your sense of identity and view of yourself. If you are unable to construct a logical narrative about your own value, say because of the structural issues you face in your life, then your executive function is going to struggle to feel good about itself. Finding a way to construct a narrative where your child feels seen and valued will help them to build back their self-esteem and start feeling good about themselves again.

Typical Struggles

The biggest self-esteem issue that children with ADHD struggle with is feeling like they are good at things. They might have trouble succeeding in, for example, an academic setting that requires them to sit still for long periods of time or focus on difficult work with lots of distractions around them. They also might struggle to be well-liked in a social context because their social behavior might be slightly out of the ordinary. They might even struggle to pick up hobbies because they can't seem to commit to the same after school activity for longer than a few weeks, always wanting to move onto the next thing. These kinds of struggles are very normal for children with ADHD, but if they are not well-aware of the commonality of these struggles, then they might feel really alone. In the next section, we will look at how you can set up support systems in your child's life to help them overcome these self-esteem issues.

How to Help

There are two key areas in which you should invest to help your child with their self-esteem. The first is accommodations. Like it or not, your child is going to have to go through certain standardized systems in their life. If their ADHD is so severe that they really can't be in a school environment at all, then you might want to consider homeschooling options (either by yourself or a paid private tutor). However, if you think they *are* able to function in a school context, they are just struggling, then you will need to put accommodations in place. These will not only help them actually succeed, but lead to a huge boost in self-esteem. If they are suddenly able to accomplish at the same rate as their peers, then they will feel a lot more sure of themselves, creating a stronger sense of self and their own abilities. The second way in which you can meaningfully improve your child's self-esteem is through encouraging their existing abilities. Chances are, your child has something they're good at, whether that be drawing or sports or talking to adults. Whatever their talent, you should make sure to really emphasize that talent, rather than blandly assure them that they are good at everything. Children aren't stupid—they know when adults are lying to them. If you make sure to point out the things that they are really good at, they will read more authenticity into it and it will actually have a more meaningful effect on their self-esteem.

Following these techniques will help you to boost your child's self-esteem while still working with their ADHD.

CHAPTER 9:

BONDING AND COMMUNICATING

As we've stated before in this book, opening lines of communication is an essential aspect of helping your child through ADHD. If you don't understand what's going on with them, and they don't understand what you're trying to do to help, then you run the risk of lots of conflicts down the road. Making sure that you are working together is essential to the inherently collaborative process of helping your child through ADHD. If you leave them to solve their issues on their own, then they are going to feel abandoned or helpless, since you are their vital support system and their practical access to resources. But on the other hand, if you take all the matters into your own hands, your child is going to feel like they have no autonomy in their own recovery, or even possibly not know what is going on. Since they need to eventually become their own support network as they become an adult, involving them in the process is essential to helping them build skills. But it's not easy.

Chances are, if your child has undiagnosed ADHD, the two of you have had some fraught times. You've probably been frustrated with them in the past, possibly even punished them for things that you now realize were merely ADHD symptoms. If this is the case, you don't have to worry: You didn't know what was going on. And besides, relationships can be repaired. What you need to do now that you realize what is really going on with your child is to construct a clear line of communication as well as strong mutual trust. In this chapter, we will discuss the building of these relationships and instruct you on how to do so. First, we will look at the important benefits of constructing this strong relationship with your child, listing some of the most important emotional benefits. Then, we will talk about the importance of honesty in your communication, especially how your own honesty factors in as a model. Finally, we will talk about communication strategies that can have a meaningful effect on you and your child's relationship, helping you to repair some emotional damage and create a strong, long-lasting relationship going forward.

The Importance of Creating a Strong Relationship

The value of creating a meaningful connection between you and your child cannot be overstated. One of the biggest mistakes parents make is assuming that their relationship is strong just because of blood ties. You assume that, because they're your child, you will always have an emotional bond with them. But this is not necessarily the case. Just like marriages and friendships, parent and child relationships need work in order to thrive. If you have a difficult relationship with your child, then you need to approach it in the same way as if your marriage was rocky: put emotional effort in. Children are complex people with intricate feelings, grudges, secrets, and aspirations just like you, so you need to approach them in as complex a way as you would with other adults. They deserve this kind of treatment. If you make that a priority in your life, then you will really see the benefits. Your child will start trusting you more, rely on you more closely for help, and start to build a close bond. In this section, we will talk about some of the most important aspects and benefits of creating that emotional bond between you and your child and opening up lines of communication.

Unconditional Love

In the family context, and sometimes outside, there is a concept called "unconditional love." Unconditional love is essentially a type of love that is not put into jeopardy by any personal failings, be they academic, financial, or sometimes even moral. Think of the typical phrase used in wedding vows: "For richer or for poorer, in sickness and in health, etc." This is describing the unconditional love members of the same family unit are supposed to feel for one another. But unconditional love is somewhat nuanced. On one hand, there are a lot of family dynamics wherein love is conditional. Parents who become emotionally unavailable when their children disappoint them academically or when they don't go into the field they imagined for them, are not demonstrating unconditional love. So just because you are related to someone does not mean that you are actually practicing unconditional love. On the other hand, you can easily mistake unconditional love with blind love. Despite its name, unconditional love does have some conditions. However, those conditions are about violating the contract of the relationship, not about who you are individually. So, betraying you or cutting you out of your life doesn't necessarily mean you have to keep loving them, but them making choices that you don't necessarily agree with, but which aren't putting their life at risk, means you still have to show them care. So, when practicing unconditional love with your child, make sure that you enforce the importance of mutual care, but still make it clear that everyone can be themselves, or fail at things, and they will still be loved.

How to Work on This

Working on your unconditional love with your child is all about acceptance. You accept them, but also they accept you. This is why being willing to admit that you're not a perfect person or parent is essential. Being able to admit when you've done wrong, or apologize to your child, is one of the biggest things you can do as a parent. Not only does it give you accountability and help your child feel heard when they criticize you, but it also helps you to show them that anyone can make mistakes. If you act like you're the perfect parent all the time and make out like you can do no wrong, then your child is probably going to fear that they can't make any mistakes or fear you thinking badly of them. Admitting your mistakes is saying: "Hey, I messed up, and that's okay, so if you mess up sometimes, that's okay too." For kids with ADHD, who probably feel like they're constantly making mistakes and being told that they're wrong, this can be a really reassuring thing to hear.

You also need to get straight the difference between things that are harmful and things that you don't agree with. Your child wanting to play team sports when you are more of a bookish family is not the end of the world, but finding out that they've been experimenting with drugs is cause for concern. Them choosing to go to community college for graphic design instead of an ivy league school for business is their personal choice, while them wanting to stay out all night with strangers is a concern. The difference between these two things is that the former is something that people do in general that is not objectively harmful, whereas the latter is something that might jeopardize their personal safety. Chances are, your child is going to do something in their life that you don't agree with, but if it is not going to cause them immediate harm, it's best to let them try their best and love them unconditionally through it.

Bringing You Closer Together as a Family

If two people in a family unit are experiencing difficulties, then the entire family suffers. If you and your child with ADHD are constantly at odds with one another, this has a strong effect on your relationship with anyone else in your family, such as your spouse, parents, or other children. In order to keep the family unit strong, everyone has to find a way to connect with one another and see eye-to-eye. Repairing any struggles you might have with your child with ADHD is an integral way in which you can improve the dynamics of your family closer together. Improve your relationship with your other children or other members of your family by building a stronger connection to your ADHD child and trying to diffuse potential tension within your relationship.

What You Might Be Doing Wrong

Unfortunately, no one is a perfect parent. We scream sometimes, we forget things, we're too tired to take our kids somewhere—it's all normal. There's no shame in admitting to doing something wrong on occasion. When it comes to unconditional love, there's a chance you might be giving either too much or too little. If you are giving too much, then you might be going too easy on your child. You might be giving them support even when they are acting in a way that needs reeling them in. This might sound like being kind, but you are actually not doing your child any favors. Children tend to toe the line, and it is your job as a parent to be clear about where that line is, otherwise your child will see fit to break the rules whenever they want.

However, you might also not be giving them enough, withholding affection when they disappoint you or don't act in the way you want. If you behave in a way that makes it seem as though your child is no longer special to you if they, say, fail a math test, can be really damaging. Your child can start to feel like your love for them is conditional and only based on their superficial abilities, not their innate qualities. Children need to feel like you love them for them, not for the things they do, so make

181

sure that even when you reprimand them for something they are doing, that you also make it clear that you still love them, you just want them to succeed. If you are not striking a balance between these two things, you are likely going to have a problem with your child.

How to Work on This

One of the most important ways to start mitigating conflict between you and your ADHD child is to choose your battles. Not everything they do is going to be alright with you, or even good with them, but sometimes it's better to let things slide than get into conflicts over every single little thing. For example, if you have already had a tension-filled day and your other children really want to spend time with you, but your child with ADHD just can't seem to finish their homework, you can afford to let it slide one night for the sake of the family dynamic. Of course, you shouldn't do this every single night of the week, but if it just becomes too much on occasion, don't be afraid to just choose peace over winning. The other thing you can do is try to outsource some of the discipline so you don't *always* have to be the bad guy. If you can afford it, put your child in tutoring a couple of times a week. This means that someone else is making sure they are doing their homework—at an appointed time—and you can focus on other things. Doing something like this can often actually have a huge liberating effect on the family. Suddenly, homework time, the site of many legendary battles, is no longer an issue and everyone feels the burden lifted. Taking the time to really prioritize family over making sure your child does *everything* right can really diffuse a lot of tension in your relationship with them as well as the rest of your family.

Two Heads Are Better Than One

Like we said in the introduction to this chapter, recovering from ADHD and even simply receiving any treatment or accommodations for the condition can be a very daunting practice. You and your child will have to go through a serious period of adjustment and searching when you are starting out, so having both of you connected in trying to solve it is a great asset. Since everyone's ADHD journey is different, you should be making sure that your child has ample opportunity to give their input. A strategy you might have heard online might work for one child, but it won't necessarily work for yours. The only way to really know whether something is working for your child is to really deeply consult with them and make sure that they feel comfortable sharing with you. This is truly one of the most important parts of the process—that your child is comfortable. If you set up an intimidating or hierarchical relationship with them, then you won't get very far. They will always feel like they can't fully share how they feel with you and might hesitate to speak out if they feel like a strategy isn't really helping them. It's important to be very receptive to their feedback during these kinds of conversations so that they know they can always be honest with you in the future. Opening up lines of communication not only helps to build a bond with your child, but also helps to better customize their ADHD treatment going forward.

What You Might Be Doing Wrong

Being collaborative is difficult at the best of times. And when you have a small child, they are not necessarily the best of collaborators. You might not feel like they know what they want or are very diligent about what they can handle. You might be concerned that they are too young to really contribute to their own ADHD plan, but this actually isn't true. Even if you have a really little kid, they are still able to judge whether or not they are enjoying something or whether it is difficult for them. If your child is old enough to have identifiable ADHD, then they are old enough to have a say in how it is treated. Micromanaging too much, and always dictating what your child does without consulting them can make them feel really frustrated. Remember: your child is the one living with the condition, you are there to be their facilitator. All you have to do is be their connector to the services they need, research the condition for them, and offer support. You might have all the research down, but you can't see inside your child's head and therefore don't always know what's best for them. If you want to have a strong relationship, let them collaborate with you.

How to Work on This

Back in Chapter 3, we talked about how important it is to make your child's ADHD recovery journey something inherently customizable. They won't be able to have too much of a say in the way ADHD affects them, but it can be a real gift to be able to have a say in the way they are accommodated for it. However, they are likely not going to be as well-educated about possible ADHD treatments and accommodations as, say, a medical professional or even just an adult who is able to research more easily. So, they can't exactly come to you with the kind of accommodations or treatments they might think they need. However, your child will be able to tell if something isn't working for them. If you try a technique from this book or from other literature on ADHD and your child just doesn't seem to be responding to it, don't try to force it. Take the cue that this isn't a technique they particularly respond to and try something else. If you are skilled at making them feel heard and understood, then they should start to develop the skills to help them communicate that to you.

In the interest of time, and your child's comfort, it is almost always good to drop something that isn't working. Bear in mind, though, that some habits take a while to form and you might not be able to fully understand the benefits unless you've kept at it for a while. But as always, if you've been trying for weeks, or it is causing lots of fights, it's probably best to move onto other techniques that might be less tension-inducing.

Building Their Emotional Intelligence

Emotional intelligence is one of the most important qualities we develop throughout adulthood. Of course, like many other skills, many adults struggle deeply to develop this skill, not putting in the effort or having someone to teach them. But if you are a responsible parent, you have the power to make sure that your child does not become one of these people. By building a strong connection with them early in life, you are modeling emotional skills that they will carry with them through their life. If the seeds of emotional intelligence are planted now, then your child will have a much easier time adjusting to the complex emotional world of adulthood. Engaging in emotional repression throughout childhood not only delays the development of these essential skills, but also causes the active thwarting of these skills. Repression is the enemy of emotional intelligence and makes your child feel ashamed of their emotions rather than inclined to investigate them. Teaching these skills — communication, listening, and emotional care — will not only help you cultivate a good relationship with your child now, but will also help them down the road.

What You Might Be Doing Wrong

We've all had experiences that have emotionally stunted us, and not everyone received the kind of emotional support or education they needed when they were a kid. If you don't feel like you're the most emotionally intelligent person in the world, then you are probably going to have a pretty hard time raising a child with ADHD. If you don't have these skills in place, there are likely going to be times when you unload your own emotional baggage on your child, or at least let it affect your judgment. Maybe you felt like teachers never understood you, so you unload that emotional pain onto your child. It's good to get support, but your child doesn't know how to do that for you yet. You need to find other people in your life to help you with that support. Having lots of unresolved issues, especially ones that pertain to any aspect of your child's ADHD journey means that you are going to have a really difficult time helping them through theirs.

How to Work on This

Teaching emotional intelligence starts with modeling it yourself. Kids learn by modeling, and so kids who grow up with parents who are repressed don't learn the kinds of emotional skills they will need later on in life. Therefore, as a parent you need to learn to develop your own emotional intelligence to help your child through their difficulties. This might mean going to therapy yourself—even if you don't think you need it—to learn more about who you are. Short of that, you could start journaling, trying to have deeper conversations with friends, or just generally start to refine your emotional skills. Then, when you come back to your child, you will be better informed and be able to help them more easily. When they see you modeling these more emotionally-attuned qualities, it will make them see that these are signs of adulthood, strength, and intelligence. They will also be able to imitate your behavior to help them learn in more depth about the ways in which to practice emotional intelligence. Helping your child to see the way towards emotional intelligence through modeling is very important.

Authenticity and Honesty

Offering support is all very well, but if it isn't coming from a place of honesty, then your child is probably not going to benefit from it as much. Similarly, if your child does not feel like they can be honest with you, then they are not going to be as comfortable sharing how they feel with you and thus won't let you know when they are not feeling good or having trouble. For these reasons, fostering a culture of honesty among the two of you is one of the most important things you can do for your child during their ADHD journey. They will feel more comfortable with you, you will understand one another better, and the whole relationship between the two of you will feel distinctly unique. In this section, we are going to talk about the importance, as well as the process of fostering honesty between you and your child with ADHD. First, we are going to talk about the importance of "judgment-free zones" which can do wonders for the sense of camaraderie between you and your child and save the both of you a lot of shame. Next, we will talk about the dual nature of honesty and how you need to work on your ability to be honest with your child as well as their ability to be honest with you. And finally, we will talk about the importance of individual expression as it pertains to honesty—we all get to be ourselves. These modules will help you to construct a more honest connection with your child.

Judgement-Free Zones

What's the #1 reason that we all tend to feel scared of sharing things with others? Because we fear judgment. Our innate sense of shame tends to overtake our desire to know and be known by others. When we fear that we might be judged, that feeling we want to share suddenly seems that much more embarrassing and we recoil. Sometimes it is worse between parents and children.

Parents worry that their children won't see them as good role models if they admit wrongdoing or say something embarrassing. Children, conversely, think that their parents might punish them if they admit to feeling a certain way or doing something wrong. Sometimes, these fears are founded, but it doesn't have to be this way. One strategy you can implement between you and your child for fostering more clear honesty is the "judgment free zone." This is a way that you can eliminate any judgment between you and your child for a certain conversation. Here, we will talk about this method and its ins and outs.

How It Works

So how exactly do you practice the "judgment-free zones"? What do they consist of? Well, part of that is up to you. There are two main ways to carry out this practice. The first is to create areas, or even signals (such as a talking stick, bear, etc.) that signify that you're in a judgment-free zone. Your child (or you!) can step into this judgment-free zone in order to confess something that they don't want to be judged or punished for and the rule is that everyone has to listen with respect and agree not to judge. Of course, you want to avoid your child abusing this, and obviously if they confess something very serious that you do think they should be reprimanded for, you can bend the rules, but if it is something minor, like staying up late on their iPad or forgetting to hand in an assignment, you should respect the rules. The second way to go about this is to create fixed times throughout the week where you engage in honesty and no-judgment attitudes. Maybe it's every Monday night after school, and you and your child sit down with a snack and say that you can confess to one thing each. You sharing that you forgot to put in the laundry yesterday or have been slacking on work a little bit this week will make your child a lot more comfortable sharing some of their mistakes or shortcomings to you. If neither of you has anything to confess from that week, maybe think of something from a long time ago so no one has to feel like the odd one out. Both of these techniques help you and your child to confess important things that maybe neither of you would have admitted to otherwise. That is how you build honesty and authenticity!

It Goes Both Ways

Jumping off from the last section, an integral thing to remember when you are trying to closely bond with your child is that authenticity and communication goes both ways. You might feel constantly frustrated that your child is not confessing things to you enough, but that isn't fair unless you are also being honest with them. And being honest doesn't just mean admitting to your faults like we talked about in the "judgment-free zone," it also means keeping your child on the same page as you when it comes to plans and especially circumstances around their accommodations and treatment. If they feel like you are keeping things from them or that they don't have a say in what they are doing, then this means that they are going to be less likely to be open with you. Opening lines of communication thus means much more than just "getting your child to talk," it means opening up a two-way street of communication from which your child can stand to gain a lot as well. Making sure that you are being as honest with your child as they are being with you is one of the keys to a successful relationship between the two of you.

Free to Be You and Me

Everyone is different. We all have our likes and dislikes, our little quirks that make us who we are. When we are close with others, we might tend to clash over these things. You might not always see eye-to-eye with your child, especially because their ADHD symptoms might cause outbursts or niche, hyper focused interests that you don't share.

Hyper Fixations are very common in neurodivergent people. They could be a TV show, a creative form, or even a period in history or a discipline in science. At worst, they can blind your child to other opportunities for learning, especially if they are, say, watching nothing but the same movie over and over. But most of the time, they are very harmless and can actually bestow your child with a lot of niche and interesting knowledge that not a lot of other people know. It might be tempting to be dismissive of these things, or at least indifferent towards them, but this can actually be very hurtful to a child. As much as they might broadcast the things they are interested in, they are likely still insecure about them and if you as their parents insult or belittle them in any way, it could really hurt them.

One thing that you could try to do is show a really vested interest in something that your child likes, especially if it is a hyperfixation. Watch their favorite movie with them and talk about it with them enthusiastically afterwards. Offer to proofread their comic book they've been working on, or to take them to a convention for their favorite sci-fi show. In turn, you could let them in on something you really love. Show them an old movie (that is appropriate, of course) or take them on a trip to a city you traveled to when you were young. Sharing in each others' interests will broaden both of your horizons and help you to understand the other more, not to mention flexing your open mindedness muscles! Acknowledging and celebrating each of your uniqueness can be a great opportunity for bonding and growth.

Your Role as a Communicator

For the second part of this chapter, we will be talking about communication, and more importantly, communication skills. We all think that we are good communicators, or at least that communication is somewhat easy. We like to think that we know how to articulate ourselves very well. But the truth is that communication is actually very hard. It takes a lot of work to learn how to articulate yourself properly, and even more work to learn how to articulate yourself properly to certain specific people. People go to university for years to study the complex minutiae of writing or even linguistics. These things are far from simplistic. You can always benefit from working on your communication skills. Whether it's for work, for your creative pursuits, or for your relationships, especially relationships with your children, who haven't learned communication skills yet. This is the most important point: Because your child is still getting a grasp on language, they are far from being a sophisticated, articulate adult. Thus, you have to be twice as good a communicator to open those lines with your child. You are also teaching them communication skills through this modeling, meaning that you also have to make sure all your communication skills are well-in-checked. Here, we will look at six basic communication strategies that you can use to improve your relationship with your child.

Communication Strategy #1: Listening

It might sound counter-intuitive, but actually the most important thing about communicating is the ability to listen. As the parent of a child with ADHD, you are probably always frustrated with your child not listening to you and even ignoring what you say when they *do* listen to you. This can be a really frustrating experience for parents, but what you have to remember is that you need to listen too. Sometimes when you are angry that your child isn't listening, it's because they have something to tell you and can't wait until you are done. Having the patience to maybe listen to them first will help you to connect with them and to show them that they are important. Sometimes, if you just let them say what they want to say, or even interrupt you a few times, they will actually then be more receptive to what you want to say to them. Your child also might be going through something difficult that is making it hard for them to pay attention. Sometimes, if you allow them to say what's going on with them first, it can help you to change your communication style to fit their current mental state. And finally, good listening is just a great thing to model for your child. If they never observe you listening, then how are they supposed to know how to listen? Making sure that they understand what listening entails is a very important thing to do for your child. And for someone with ADHD, who likely struggles with listening, it is this modeling that will help them to better develop that skill in their life.

Bonus: Active Listening

One particular brand of listening that is really important to understand is "active listening." So what is the difference between "active listening" and "passive listening"? Well, active listening involves communicating to the person you are listening to that you are listening, rather than just blankly staring at them. Some active listening strategies can be, for example, nodding while someone is speaking, repeating what they said back to them, or making sure to very closely connect the next thing you say to that person's point. All these strategies will be noticed by the speaker, making them feel like you truly connected with and understood what they were saying. If you want to be a top-tier listener, then you should make sure that you practice your active listening skills in particular. Modeling these active listening skills to your child is also a good way to improve their listening skills.

Communication Strategy #2: The 'I' Statement

One of the biggest barriers to communication is the feeling of being attacked. When people feel they are being accused of something, they tend to tense up, become defensive, and generally shut down. If you approach a difficult conversation with your child as if it is a big accusation game, then they are going to start to go on the defensive and not share anything with you. Instead, what you should do is use 'I' statements rather than 'you' statements. 'I' statements focus on how you are feeling about the situation, whereas 'you' statements accuse the other person of doing something. What the 'I' statement does is it takes the focus off the intentions of the other person and puts the focus on the impact of their actions. They might not think that they have done anything wrong, or intended to do anything wrong, but upon seeing the impact of their actions, might be more inclined to listen. When you hear "you did something wrong," your immediate reaction is to defend yourself. On the other hand, when you hear someone say "that thing you did hurt my feelings," you're probably more likely to feel bad and apologize. Since you can't deny another person's feelings, the 'I' statement is much harder to dispute. This helps open up the conversation and mitigate any feelings of accusation.

Let's take a possible scenario in which you could use either an 'I' statement or a 'you' statement. Let's say you have an 11 year old with ADHD who walks to school by herself. She has a phone and you like for her to text you before she leaves school so you know when she's walking home and can watch for her. But she always seems to forget, leaving you worried every day. A 'you' statement would look like this: "You always forget to text me when you leave school, you're so negligent." Immediately, your daughter is going to be on the defensive, not wanting to be called negligent. Instead, you could say something like: "It's my job to take care of you and it really makes me very anxious when I don't hear from you. I know you might think it's silly, but would you mind trying a bit harder to remember so that I can rest a little easier?" By explaining your side of the story and focusing on the emotional impact of the actions, you are taking the accusation off your daughter and instead reminding her why the rule is there in the first place. The second statement is much more likely to get a positive response from her and is therefore the more effective parenting strategy.

Communication Strategy #3: Have Goals in Mind

If you are initiating a conversation with your child, you should know what you want to get out of that conversation. If you aren't sure why you are bringing something up, then you probably want to take a longer look at why you are starting this conversation in the first place. If you reflect further, you might find that it actually isn't strictly necessary to bring up. Or, you might find a more focused way of doing so. When confronting your child about something they have done, you never want to approach it with shame, but instead with the goal of growth. Children mess up all the time and so you need to choose your battles wisely. Chastising them over something they can't change won't be very productive, unless the goal of the conversation is to make sure they never do it again. Thus, the goal should be something concrete for the future, and hopefully something productive, rather than negative.

So, let's say for example, your child's grades are slipping. You are worried about this and so you try to confront them. If you don't have clear, constructive goals in mind, you run the risk of simply making them feel bad about their academic performance and getting nowhere. But if you go into the conversation with the goal of: "Let's find out what is causing these slipping grades," or "Let's discover a type of support that might help them get their grades back up," then you will likely have a much more clear and productive conversation. You will also likely be approaching your child in a far less accusatory way. They will be more likely to cooperate with you for this reason as well. Making sure you have a clear goal in mind will focus the conversation and keep it moving towards a more productive goal.

Communication Strategy #4: Be Comfortable With Leaving Things Open

That being said, there is absolutely no obligation to solve all of your child's issues in one fell swoop. It is likely that there is a lot to talk about with any given topic and so there is no obligation to figure everything out at once. Just because you have a goal going into the conversation doesn't mean that you necessarily have to accomplish it that day. You can think of your conversation as being part one of many that will eventually lead you towards your goal. One thing that can be helpful is to set smaller goals within your larger goals. For example, in the grades scenario, you might not be able to solve the major problems right away, such as establishing the kinds of support your child might need to improve their grades. Instead, the first conversation could just be diagnostic, trying to establish that there is a problem, or that your child wants any help in the first place. Having these smaller goals-within-goals can really make a difference in your child's ability to get through these conversations and still feel accomplished at the end. So if you sit down and don't hash it all out at once, don't worry! You can always come back to it.

Communication Strategy #5: Don't Be Afraid to Take Space

Along the same lines, communication can be really tiring. This is especially true for children with ADHD, who might struggle to pay attention to a long conversation or even just sit still for a long period of time. If you and your child are talking about a really serious topic, it is likely that it is very emotionally draining for them. They might feel like they can't take it or get tired very quickly. There

200

is no shame in taking a small break—even as short as ten minutes—and resuming the conversation. Going to the bathroom, having a glass of juice, or even going on a small walk around the block can really clear your head and make you feel refreshed enough to come back to the conversation with fresh eyes. You might even want to follow the age-old advice and "sleep on it" if you are facing a particularly difficult decision. When it comes to hashing out a long and complicated issue, it is always fair to take breaks and can even improve your concentration.

Communication Strategy #6: Understand What They Understand

One of the biggest mistakes people can make in communicating, especially communicating with children, is not realizing when someone doesn't understand what you're saying. If you're using a word your child doesn't know or trying to gloss over something complicated, you might lose them and then the entire purpose of your communication is moot. During your conversation, you should make sure that the both of you are always on the same page, frequently checking in on whether your child is actually following all of what you are saying. This way, you will make sure that they never lose track of what you are talking about and the communication will be strong and effective.

CHAPTER 10:

ADHD IS A SUPERPOWER

Thus far throughout this book, we have talked almost exclusively about the negative consequences ADHD can have on your child's life. We've talked about the limitations, the setbacks, the things that make your child have a more difficult time than others. However, there is a whole other side to ADHD that is separate from all those negative things. In fact, there are things about ADHD that can actually make it a superpower!

Many children with ADHD have exceptional abilities that mean they can do things other children can't, and even have completely unique experiences. For the last chapter in this book, we are going to focus on these positive aspects of ADHD that mean your child truly has unique qualities. First, we will talk about how powerful accepting your child can really be when it comes to adjusting to their ADHD diagnosis, exploring the relationship between acceptance from others and acceptance from the self. Next, we will look at some of the particular natural strengths that come along with ADHD and the ways in which they might benefit your child through their life. And finally, we will talk about some techniques your child can implement in order to more efficiently take advantage of these strengths. By the end of this chapter, you should be a lot more comfortable with the idea of your child having ADHD and be more understanding of the amazing things your child really is capable of!

The Power of Acceptance

We all want to be accepted and accept ourselves. One of the basic human needs is to feel like you are a good and worthwhile person, and to know that others believe so as well. This, however, can be a hard thing to grapple with if you have a diagnosis like ADHD, which can really throw off your ability to feel like you are a worthwhile person. However, with the aid of others and a lot of self-acceptance, you can begin on that journey. Your child likely has some serious self-esteem issues in relation to their ADHD, meaning that their self acceptance is fairly low. They might even be facing lack of acceptance from people in their life, from teachers to peers to extended family members. Both of these things can be devastating to your child's sense of self and belief in their own abilities. If you want your child to have a good and accepting relationship with their ADHD, then you should be helping them work hard on their self acceptance and in turn, working on your own acceptance of them. In this section, we will look at these two kinds of acceptance and talk about how they are strictly necessary for someone to begin healing on their ADHD journey as well as take advantage of some of the perks.

Acceptance From Others

It might not be fashionable to admit it, but acceptance from others actually has a strong impact on our self-esteem as people. We want to feel like we are part of a community, that other people think well of us. This is just part of human nature. For children in particular, feeling like they have acceptance from their parents is actually a very integral thing. Feeling like your parents don't really accept you or like who you are can be really devastating to a child. So the first step towards making sure that your child feels accepted in the world is to do so yourself.

But what does this look like? How do you make sure your child knows you accept them and their ADHD diagnosis? One of the best ways you can do this is to never deny that they have ADHD. Be loud and proud about it. Don't act like the condition has any sort of shame or stigma attached to it — simply be open and calm about it. Even if you have some lingering stigma about the condition, make sure that you deal with that yourself and don't involve your child in it. Another thing you can do is to make sure that you acknowledge your child's qualities that exist outside of their ADHD. ADHD might be a very serious condition that changes the way your brain works, but it also is just one part of your child's personality. Highlighting who they are outside of their ADHD can really help them to construct a narrative about who they are that is both comfortable with their ADHD diagnosis, but also conscious of their unique self outside of that will put them on the path towards self acceptance.

Acceptance From the Self

Having acceptance from others is very helpful, but it is also important that this acceptance translates into acceptance from yourself. Failing to really accept who you are and being comfortable in your own skin is a really terrible state to be in. Unfortunately, many children don't have the emotional tools to really coach themselves into self acceptance. This means that you are going to have to do a large portion of the work yourself to make sure that your child has the emotional tools to start accepting themselves. First, you need to get a sense of where they are in their self acceptance. Sit down and talk to them about how they feel about themselves. You can even give them a self-reflexive activity to work on if you are worried that they aren't going to be able to express themselves in words. Get a sense of how they are—do they feel really bad about themselves? Are they being really self-deprecating? Do they value their abilities very low? If this is the case then they definitely need to work on their acceptance of themselves.

Modeling is very important here. You are already modeling being accepting of them through practicing it yourself, but there is also another type of modeling, which is modeling self acceptance yourself. You might think it's harmless to say self-deprecating things about yourself all the time or insult yourself, but it can actually have a highly negative impact on your children. They see you do this and they think that it's the only way to be. They don't understand that these things are a joke or that you don't really mean them. One study traced the effects of negative self-talk in adults on children, in this case in relation to dieting. They found that parents talking negatively about their own weight increased the likelihood of their child developing an eating disorder (Jones, 2020). From this example, we can see how this kind of negative self-talk can really impact the way children see themselves. So if you want your child to have better self-esteem and higher self acceptance, make sure that you don't badmouth yourself in front of them either. Highlighting their strengths, which we will talk about in the next section, is another important tactic.

Highlighting the Strengths of ADHD

From all the symptoms and potentially negative consequences of ADHD we have talked about throughout this book, it might be hard to believe that there are any positives. But rest assured: There are plenty of things your child might have that make them better-suited to certain activities or pursuits. The neurodivergent brain has the advantage of looking at the world a little differently than everyone else. It is capable of creating a fresh take on the world and learning in a way people never thought was possible. This is what is sometimes known as a "left hand advantage" or "negative-frequency-dependent selection." AKA a unique trait that is made useful by the fact that it is unique. Some researchers believe that the reason there are left-handed people in the world is because the rarity of left handedness is an advantage in fighting and sports (Llaurens et al., 2008). The average person is less experienced at fighting a left handed person or pitching to a left handed batter. Thus, left handedness persists as something useful, but only if it remains unique, thus never exceeding the 10–15% mark. Neurodivergence could be seen as similar—a different type of brain that is useful insofar as it is unique. You can think of your child in this way: They have a perspective that is less common and thus they provide an advantage to things like research, conversation, and creativity. Here, we will look at some of the best benefits to having ADHD and how it can actually give you an edge in life.

Strength #1: Hyperfocusing

As we've talked about earlier in this book, people with ADHD have an uncanny ability to hyperfocus on things. They are able to sit down with a task and not take their attention off of it for hours. Now, sometimes this can prevent problems, like forgetting to do other important tasks, but from a different perspective, it is a highly-beneficial thing. Children who have the ability to hyperfocus can create amazing things. They might spend hours in their room writing stories that help them build the skills required to become a professional writer one day. Or they might spend an entire weekend learning an instrument, teaching themselves basic guitar chords in a matter of hours. Or they might come home every day after school and just run soccer drills in the backyard. These tendencies might be a bit annoying, but step back and realize that your child has actually accomplished something amazing. The trick is to be able to control when your child hyperfocuses. Through ADHD training, they can perhaps gain a stronger control over their focus, but you don't want them to lose this hyperfocusing quality forever. In fact, it can actually be one of their greatest assets.

Strength #2: Fresh Perspective

Like we said in the introduction to this section, people with ADHD offer a different perspective on the world. We're used to conversations with, and media created by, neurotypical people, which means it is going to have a particular way of looking at the world. It is going to have the conventional attention span, structure, and the same way of feeling about things in general. This can get boring after a while. After all: Art is about exploring other people with experiences different from our own. It is able to broaden our perspective on the human experience and help us learn about how other people think through creative expression. If everyone who created art was the same, then there would be no reason to keep making things. People with ADHD can make art that is unique and beautiful while also educating people on the issue of neurodivergence. And it's not just art! Researchers who study scientific or historical topics can also benefit from the help of neurodivergent people who can provide them with a fresh perspective on things they might have previously overlooked. When your child with ADHD contributes their perspective, it will help them go far in the world and people will certainly thank them for it.

Strength #3: Spontaneous Personality

Due to their incredibly changeable natures, people with ADHD tend to be really spontaneous. Of course, this can be a challenge when they seem to float from task to task, but it can also mean that they have really interesting ideas at the spur of the moment. Going on a trip or having a party with someone with ADHD can be really fun. There's a strong likelihood that your child is known as the fun kid on the playground, the one who always comes up with all the interesting games for the other kids to play. This quality means that your kid is imaginative, interesting, and enjoyable to be around! Just make sure that they know when to reel in their spontaneity and not abandon important things.

Strength #4: Courageous Tendencies

Besides being highly spontaneous, people with ADHD are very often courageous. They are more apt to take risks. You could look at this as an aversion to consequences, but if you see it from a more positive perspective, you will realize that there is actually a really great side of this. Your child might be more inclined than other children to try riding a bike for the first time or dive headfirst into a new skill. These qualities mean that your child is very unlikely to miss out on joys in life, always learning new things and seeking out new opportunities. They will possibly not have the same petty fears that other people do about trying new things, but be bold and willing to risk it all for something truly exciting.

Strength #5: Confidence

Despite some of the self-esteem issues that can be commonplace in someone with ADHD, there is also an innate confidence that comes along with the condition. Talking over people, moving onto new things when they see fit, and the like can all be seen as expressions of immense confidence. If your child is able to overcome some of the shame and stigma that tends to be associated with people with ADHD, then they will be able to access a higher confidence that is unparalleled. They will certainly go far with that kind of attitude, being able to have certainty in their abilities.

How to Take Advantage of These Strengths

All of these strengths are all very well, but you actually have to know how to make use of them if you are going to have any luck. When your child is undergoing ADHD treatment, it is of course important for them to try to manage their symptoms, but it is also important for them to try to tap into their innate strengths. Instead of only focusing on the negatives of having an ADHD brain, they should try to reach further and find all the great things that they can do with it. But this is easier said than done. Without the right know-how, your child will just end up treating their ADHD journey like a mitigation of all their negative qualities, rather than an opportunity to cultivate truly great positive ones. In this section, we will look at some of the methods your child can use to help them really tap into their ADHD superpowers!

Method #1: Creating an ADHD-Specific Schedule

The typical schedule with the work-break-work structure is generally effective for neurotypical brains, but for someone with ADHD it can be completely unproductive. What's great about the ADHD brain is its ability to go from task to task relatively quickly, shifting gears to be in a completely different mindset within minutes. If your child really wants to tap into this amazing strength, one great thing they can do is to create a schedule that is fitting to the ADHD brain. For example, instead of one hour of homework, one hour of outdoor time, and one hour of TV time, you could instead break it into chunks of ten minutes each and go through the cycle three times. This mitigates boredom and helps your child always feel fresh, like they are never really sitting there for too long understimulated. These kinds of specialized schedules can really help your child to work with, rather than fight, the kind of brain they have.

Method #2: Try Intuitive Scheduling

Kids with ADHD are deeply intuitive and have a hard time fighting their desires to do something when they want to do it. So, it can be really hard for them to adhere to a schedule. The before schedule in Method #1 is great if they are feeling more understimulated and less focused on a particular day. But what about those days where they feel like hyper fixating? On those days, it will be very hard for them to oscillate between these different tasks at a breakneck speed. In this case, they will need a different kind of schedule. One thing you can do is create two or three different kinds of schedules for a typical day—making sure that they all include necessities like mealtimes, homework, and exercise—and ask your child which one they prefer to follow on a given day. This is a great technique because it promotes choice on your child's part and helps them exercise their internal intuition while also making sure that they are able to follow the kind of schedule that works for them that day. Try out this technique and see whether your child has an easier time adhering to their schedule.

Method #3: Create an Activities Room

For children with ADHD, inspiration is going to strike at any moment. And there's nothing worse than being inspired to write something when you don't have a pen, or to paint something when you don't have a brush. For those days when your child is going to be home all Saturday hanging around, you should make sure that they have access to all the things they might need. Keep an art station, a reading nook, and a shed full of sports equipment for when your child feels like trying these things out. On days when they're supposed to be in school and they go between all these things, it can be a problem, but for these days of free time, you should encourage it! Through all these techniques, you can help your child get the most out of their ADHD and spend their treatment working with their brain style, not trying to fight it.

CONCLUSION

Raising a child with ADHD is not easy. Likely you have had some really rough times, some major fights, and a lot of disagreements. But it is also an opportunity. It is an opportunity for growth, for you to become closer to your child, and for both of you to learn more about the amazingly unique ways our brains work. If you have made it to the end of this book, you have been through a lot. You've likely come across some passages that were relatable to you—perhaps some of them a little too relatable—and read some things that have really resonated on a personal level. It might have been hard to read at parts, reminding you of some of the more fraught times between you and your child, but it has also likely given you hope that there is a better future ahead for you and your child. There are ways for them to seek treatment for their ADHD, for this treatment to lead to a much more productive and fulfilling life for your child, and most importantly, for them to be able to see their condition as a strength, not a weakness. Hopefully, you have come out of your reading experience with lots of ideas for the future of how you are going to help your child going forward.

So what are the most important things we have learned? Well, one of the most important is surely the five pillars of ADHD treatment: acceptance, emotional regulation, connection, and self-esteem. These five skills have been woven throughout the book, helping you to see the ways in which your child can truly improve their situation. Let's go back over these five points and discuss how they relate to many other parts of the book.

Acceptance is everything when it comes to the process of diagnosis. Many parents want to deny that their child has ADHD, but that won't get you anywhere. Only by truly accepting who your child is can you really start to move forward and see some improvement. We talked about acceptance in Chapter 1 when we talked about the initial process of getting diagnosed. We talked about how important it is to be able to recognize and accept ADHD symptoms in your child, especially those more specific symptoms that might be unique to their personality. We also talked about acceptance in Chapter 3, when we talked about creating a more specific experience for your own child's ADHD experience, accepting the more unique accommodations your child will need in the 'hand-made' approach. And finally, we talked about acceptance a lot in Chapter 9, where we illustrated the importance of accepting who your child really is to build that stronger emotional bond. This theme has been highly important to this book and has helped us to see the role it has in treating ADHD.

We talked about the second pillar, emotional regulation, the most in Chapter 6, where we dedicated an entire chapter to the subject. It was there where we discussed the importance of building emotional intelligence in your child. But we also talked about emotional regulation in Chapter 8, all about executive function. In this chapter, we illustrated how emotional regulation is tied up with maturity, helping you to see how important it is to teach your kids these skills. This pillar helps your child to handle the more 'explosive' aspects of their personality while building their sense of autonomy.

We discussed the third pillar—connection—the most in Chapter 9, where we discussed the importance of building a strong emotional bond with your child. But the theme of connection has run much deeper throughout this book. Connection comes up in diagnosis, in teaching scheduling skills, and in helping your child to see their ADHD superpowers for what they are. These kinds of bonds are essential for you to be able to effectively help your child through ADHD and see things from their perspective.

And finally, we focused on the qualities of the fourth pillar—self-esteem—the most in Chapters 3 and Chapter 8, which both focused on helping your child gain a sense of autonomy over their treatment. Self-esteem can really take a beating with ADHD, so it's very integral that you help your child to regulate themselves and create a caring environment towards their emotional needs. Once they know who they are and what they like about themselves, they will be able to take whatever the world throws at them.

Through these four pillars, and the many other techniques we have discussed in depth in this book, you have learned some insanely valuable skills for helping your child. You have been able to find common ground between you, fill gaps that might have previously seemed cavernous, and most importantly, given your child a way forward. If you have learned any skills from this book, we would really appreciate you leaving us a review. We love to hear the success stories from our readers and would be so grateful if you could share yours with us and the rest of the ADHD parent community. Hopefully, you will take some of these techniques and find a way to help your child through the difficult journey that is ADHD. The path is not smooth ahead, but with the right tools, you and your child can smooth it out together.

LEAVE A REVIEW

As an independent author with a small marketing budget, reviews are my livelihood on this platform. If you're enjoying this book so far, I'd really appreciate it if you left your honest feedback. I love hearing from my readers, and I personally read every single review.

REFERENCES

ADHD statistics: New ADD facts and research. (2006, October 6). ADDitude. https://www.additudemag.com/statistics-of-adhd/#:~:text=ADHD%20Prevalence%20in%20Children&text=2.4%20million%20(9.6%20percent)%20of

ADHD symptoms differ in boys and girls. (2016, March 22). Healthline. https://www.healthline.com/health/adhd/adhd-symptoms-in-girls-and-boys#Recognizing-ADHD-in-Girls

Are kids with ADHD more likely to have unhealthy habits? (n.d.). Contemporary Pediatrics. https://www.contemporarypediatrics.com/view/are-kids-adhd-more-likely-have-unhealthy-habits

Attention deficit hyperactivity disorder (ADHD) - causes. (2018, June 1). NHS. https://www.nhs.uk/conditions/attention-deficit-hyperactivity-disorder-

adhd/causes/#:~:text=ADHD%20tends%20to%20ru
n%20in

Belsky, G. (n.d.). *Executive functioning: What is executive function?* Understood.
https://www.understood.org/en/articles/what-is-executive-function

Benisek, A. (n.d.). *ADHD vs. non-ADHD brain.* WebMD.
https://www.webmd.com/add-adhd/childhood-adhd/adhd-vs-nonadhd-brain#:~:text=Studies%20of%20people%20with%20ADHD

Brain development. (n.d.). First Things First.
https://www.firstthingsfirst.org/early-childhood-matters/brain-development/#:~:text=At%20birth%2C%20the%20average%20baby%27s

CDC | Physical activity | Facts | Healthy schools. (2020, April 21). CDC.
https://www.cdc.gov/healthyschools/physicalactivity/facts.htm#:~:text=Less%20than%20one%2Dquarter%20

CHADD. (2018). *General prevalence of ADHD.* CHADD.
https://chadd.org/about-adhd/general-prevalence/

Cronkleton, E. (2021, August 13). *ADHD brain vs. normal brain: Function, differences, and more.* Medical News Today.

https://www.medicalnewstoday.com/articles/adhd
-brain-vs-normal-brain

Data and statistics about ADHD. (2021, September 23).
Centers for Disease Control and Prevention.
https://www.cdc.gov/ncbddd/adhd/data.html

Endocrine system: What is it, functions & organs. (2020,
December 5). Cleveland Clinic.
https://my.clevelandclinic.org/health/articles/2120
1-endocrine-system

Estrogen in men: Symptoms of high and low levels, and more.
(2020, November 9). Medical News Today.
https://www.medicalnewstoday.com/articles/estro
gen-in-men#symptoms-of-high-estrogen

Ferguson, L. (2017, September 22). *6 communication
strategies you need to know for your ADHD child.* Austin
Family Counseling.
https://austinfamilycounseling.com/adhd-
communication/

*5 important hormones and how they help you function: The
well for health: Health and wellness center.* (n.d.). The
Well for Health.
https://www.thewellforhealth.com/blog/5-
important-hormones-and-how-they-help-you-
function

*Five ways to help children with ADHD develop their strengths
| deborah farmer kris - intrepid ED news.* (2021, July 1).

Intrepided News. https://intrepidednews.com/five-
ways-to-help-children-with-adhd-develop-their-
strengths-deborah-farmer-kris/

Habit formation. (n.d.). Psychology Today Canada.
https://www.psychologytoday.com/ca/basics/habit
-formation

How brain chemicals influence mood and health. (2016,
September 4). UPMC HealthBeat.
https://share.upmc.com/2016/09/about-brain-
chemicals/

How common is ADHD? (2020, July 20). The Checkup.
https://www.singlecare.com/blog/news/adhd-
statistics/

*How to care for a child with ADHD: Discipline, management,
and more.* (2021, June 30). Medical News Today.
https://www.medicalnewstoday.com/articles/how-
to-care-for-a-child-with-adhd

Insulinoma. (n.d.). MedlinePlus Medical Encyclopedia.
https://medlineplus.gov/ency/article/000387.htm

Jones, G. (2020, August 18). *Parents, don't talk about weight
and dieting with your kids.* More-Love.org.
https://more-love.org/2020/08/18/parents-dont-
talk-about-weight-and-dieting-with-your-kids/

Kinman, T. (2012, December 17). *Gender differences in
ADHD symptoms.* Healthline.

https://www.healthline.com/health/adhd/adhd-
symptoms-in-girls-and-boys#Recognizing-ADHD-in-
Boys

Llaurens, V., Raymond, M., & Faurie, C. (2008). *Why are
some people left-handed? An evolutionary perspective.*
Philosophical Transactions of the Royal Society B:
Biological Sciences, 364(1519), 881–894.
https://doi.org/10.1098/rstb.2008.0235

Makowski, M., Psychologist, R. P., MacDonald, C., Dec. 1,
P. I., & 2020. (2020, December 1). *What is cognitive
flexibility and how do I help my child with it?* Foothills
Acadmeny.
https://www.foothillsacademy.org/community/arti
cles/cognitive-flexibility

McMillen, M. (n.d.). *Which children get ADHD?* WebMD.
Retrieved January 13, 2023, from
https://www.webmd.com/add-adhd/childhood-
adhd/which-children-have-adhd

Morin, A. (2019). *The 8 most effective ways to discipline a
child with ADHD.* Verywell Family.
https://www.verywellfamily.com/discipline-
strategies-for-kids-with-adhd-1094941

Myths and misunderstandings. (2018). CHADD.
https://chadd.org/about-adhd/myths-and-
misunderstandings/

Panawala, L. (2017). *Difference between hormines and neurotransmitters.* https://www.seekingbalance.com.au/wp-content/uploads/2020/08/DifferenceBetweenHormonesandNeurotransmitters_DefinitionCharacteristicsClassificationFunction.pdf

Parenting and home environment influence children's exercise and eating habits. (n.d.). ScienceDaily. Retrieved January 13, 2023, from https://www.sciencedaily.com/releases/2013/06/130618113652.htm#:~:text=FULL%20STORY-

Physical activity. (2022, October 5). World Health Organization. https://www.who.int/news-room/fact-sheets/detail/physical-activity

Porter, E. (2017, October 13). *Parenting tips for ADHD: Do's and don'ts.* Healthline. https://www.healthline.com/health/adhd/parenting-tips

Prefrontal cortex. (2018, September 17). The Science of Psychotherapy. https://www.thescienceofpsychotherapy.com/prefrontal-cortex/

Rawe, J. (n.d.). *The ADHD brain.* Understood. https://www.understood.org/en/articles/adhd-and-the-brain

Self-Soothing: What it is, benefits, & techniques to get started. (n.d.). Choosing Therapy. Retrieved January 13, 2023, from https://www.choosingtherapy.com/self-soothing/

7 foods to avoid if your child has ADHD. (n.d.). Everyday Health. https://www.everydayhealth.com/adhd-pictures/how-food-can-affect-your-childs-adhd-symptoms.aspx#:~:text=Some%20of%20the%20common%20foods

Some communication strategies for parents of kids with ADHD. (2019, November 21). The ADHD Centre. https://www.adhdcentre.co.uk/some-communication-strategies-for-parents-of-kids-with-adhd/

Symptoms - attention deficit hyperactivity disorder (ADHD). (2018). NHS. https://www.nhs.uk/conditions/attention-deficit-hyperactivity-disorder-adhd/symptoms/

Tantrums and ADHD: Causes and how to deal with them. (2021, July 9). Medical News Today. https://www.medicalnewstoday.com/articles/tantrums-and-adhd

13 parenting tips for a better home life when your kid has ADHD. (2018, August 2). Today's Parent. https://www.todaysparent.com/family/special-needs/parenting-tips-for-a-better-home-life-when-your-kid-has-adhd/

What Is ADHD? (2022). Centers for Disease Control and Prevention. https://www.cdc.gov/ncbddd/adhd/facts.html

Why is my ADHD child so angry? (2020, February 21). Start Here Parents. https://starthereparents.com/angry-adhd-child/

Why sugar is kryptonite: ADHD diet truths. (2009, October 28). ADDitude. https://www.additudemag.com/adhd-diet-nutrition-sugar/#:~:text=Foods%20rich%20in%20protein%20%E2%80%94%20lean

Williams, P. (2017, February 9). *What are the 3 types of ADHD?* ADDitude. https://www.additudemag.com/3-types-of-adhd/

Working memory - executive functioning. (n.d.). Chicago Home Tutor. Retrieved January 13, 2023, from https://chicagohometutor.com/blog/executiving-functioning-working-memory

www.ingramcontent.com/pod-product-compliance
Lightning Source LLC
Chambersburg PA
CBHW031025050325
22997CB00025B/192